SEEKING THE POSITIVES:

A Life Spent on the
Cutting Edge of Public Health

JOHN J. POTTERAT

CREATESPACE
4900 Lacross Rd., North Charleston, SC 29406, U.S.A.
A DBA of On-Demand Publishing, LLC

Cover design by John Potterat and Stephen Muth

Library of Congress Cataloging-in-Publication Data

Potterat, John J.
Seeking The Positives:
A Life Spent on the Cutting Edge of Public Health

Includes bibliographical references and Index
1. Epidemiology – Popular Works
2. Sexually Transmitted Disease – United States
I. Title

ISBN-10: 1519638183
ISBN-13: 978-1519638182

To truthniks

"My language is the common prostitute that I turn into a virgin"

—KARL KRAUS

CONTENTS

FOREWORD

"He always knew what was coming."

—Helen P. Zimmerman,

veteran STD/HIV contact tracer and clinician in Colorado Springs

In this book, John Potterat recounts a fascinating career in public health practice and research. John has been a pioneer, experimenting with disease control strategies and probing the unknown, always with scientific rigor. His record is one of prescience. Decades of John's research-based conclusions and predictions continue to be confirmed by subsequent research and experience.

This book is not simply a professional memoir. It is multiple books in one:

- a historical account of disease control in Colorado Springs;
- a partial overview and history of STD/HIV epidemiology of the last 50 years;
- a how-to manual for successful management and operation of an STD/HIV control program, or really, any organization;
- a testament to the success that can be achieved through hard work and persistence;

- an insider's perspective on the history of science in several fields in which empirical findings were dismissed, ignored, or ridiculed, but were ultimately vindicated; and

- a story of one man's remarkable career and the integrity with which he pursued it.

John was never off the job. Outside of work, in the community, John was (and is) a magnet for incidental social encounters with people whom he knew through his work. STD patients, prostitutes, pimps, and others approached John and talked with him as a trusted friend. Through his sex education presentations at schools and local media coverage of his work, many in the community knew who John was and felt comfortable approaching him with their concerns. His children tell of how, when they were growing up, pimps and prostitutes frequently called the family's home, trying to reach John, at night and on weekends.

Despite being a bootstrap operation outside of academia, the STD/HIV control program in Colorado Springs under John's leadership was for many years "Mecca" to scientists who wanted to learn about social networks underlying STD and HIV transmission. Many academic researchers came to visit John and his staff, who tutored the scientists in the basic and advanced aspects of such subjects. These researchers then went on to establish their own projects that were inspired by the examples of John and his colleagues.

John's even and diplomatic tone in this book may, in places, understate ugly realities, especially with respect to HIV/AIDS. The public health and scientific establishment has unnecessarily scared the general public in rich countries, defrauded taxpayers, denied lifesaving information to populations at risk in poor countries, and opposed scientific investigations that would allow a valid assessment of what underlies epidemics in poor countries.

In the epilogue, John describes many of the ingredients of the successes he, his staff, and colleagues achieved. These ingredients were accidents of history and characteristics of other people. He neglects to mention several of his own characteristics, many of which were undoubtedly honed during his tour of combat duty in Vietnam, that were also essential to these achievements. Throughout his career, John displayed:

- *steadfastness in the face of withering opposition* in both the scientific and community spheres;
- *ease with delegating authority* to others who demonstrated competence and backing the decisions they made;
- *a persevering and insistent manner*

   Dr. Thomas Vernon, former director of the Colorado State Department of Health, notes that "with all due credit for his intentions and admirable results, John could be brazen and pushy as hell to get there." To overcome bureaucratic inertia and competing demands on others' time, it is essential for leaders to "light a fire" under responsible individuals. John was always ready to strike a match.

- *a lack of career ambitions*

    John often described himself as a "lower government functionary with a B.A. in medieval history." He was content with that status. In his professional role, John could avoid academic researchers' trifling disputes and contests for resources and prestige.

- *zeal in spreading evidence-based information*

    John spoke out with facts about health matters in both community and scientific settings.

- *respect for and genuine curiosity about the people he served*

    As John would say, he met others "on their turf," both literally and figuratively. John and his staff spent countless evenings on the streets, in bars, and other settings educating those at greatest risk for STD and HIV. He has a keen ability to relate to people from all walks of life, due in part to his having a full life outside of work (family, friends, and hobbies) and varied life experiences prior to his work in public health. People trusted John.

- *clarity and wit in his writing*

    Dr. John Muth, former director of the health department in Colorado Springs, once jokingly described John's writing style as "flowery Frankish folderol."

- *"pleasure in finding things out,"* just as the similarly charismatic and eminent physicist Richard Feynman put it

> John's mantra was "we want to know." John is, as he says, a "truthnik" with a passion for building scientific knowledge. The research John and his staff did was not required for the routine operation of the STD/HIV control program. It simply reflected John's desire to know, and at no added cost to the public.

Other aspects of John's work environment also promoted success. He was lucky in attracting a corps of committed, talented, self-sufficient, and compassionate staff, who tolerated his ribald humor, sometimes impatient and brusque manner, and occasional short temper. This book is also *their* memoir.

John had near complete discretion in selecting and retaining staff and colleagues. Public health programs often are mired in inefficiency and mediocrity in part because managers have limited or no choices in hiring staff, and have even fewer options for removing unproductive or problematic employees.

Independence is a crucial factor in determining whether scientific research is biased. To whom are the researchers beholden? Except for a few projects funded by federal agencies, most of John's scientific work was done without funding, or, in some cases, was funded by John himself. In those few projects funded by federal agencies, John drew no salary from the grants. John had no financial vested interest in his projects, unlike nearly all researchers receiving grants. Perhaps more importantly, by not being bound to the whims of federal funding agencies (and the committees of researchers who judge what work to fund) or any other politically conflicted paymaster, John, his staff, and colleagues had freedom to pursue truth, wherever that search might lead.

John is my friend, colleague, mentor, and brother-in-scientific-arms. Many others and I are deeply grateful to John for documenting in this book the amazing string of successes and discoveries that he, his staff, and colleagues had. Enjoy the ride as he retraces his engrossing odyssey.

Devon D. Brewer, PhD

Seattle WA, May 2015

CHAPTER SUMMARIES

Prologue.   Why this book? Presents the unexpected, exceptional achievements in the epidemiology and control of various sexually transmissible diseases during four decades of active interventions by an award-winning control program. Unexpected, because achieved by public health amateurs in an obscure health department.

One.   Introduces the major intervention used: contact tracing, which consists of locating the sex partners of persons infected with STD. Contact tracing methods were enhanced by ethnography. Ethnography of an intense STD outbreak in crack cocaine gangs is detailed to illustrate this concept.

Two.   Describes the then unchartered territory of gonorrhea epidemiology and control during this epidemic, which lasted almost two decades. Details the control successes and contributions to epidemiologic science, which had implications for both national and international STD control initiatives. Substantial reductions in the gonorrhea burden using contact tracing were rigorously documented (twice) and, importantly, gonorrhea was shown to be a social disease.

Three. Being there at the beginning of the AIDS epidemic provided opportunity to blaze new trails, such as implementation of routine HIV reporting and contact tracing. Both approaches had generally been discouraged. Precise documentation of this epidemic yielded, among other notable accomplishments, a unique achievement: tracing an HIV epidemic to its very beginning. Contact tracing information acted as an epidemiologic Hubble Telescope to look back in time and observe the Big HIV Bang locally. No other published reports have provided the breadth and depth of detail obtained to elucidate the trajectory of this epidemic in a single community over a long period.

Four. New tests for chlamydia (gonorrhea's "fraternal twin") provided the opportunity to use contact tracing to control and study its community dynamics. Over time, increasingly intensive contact tracing not only occasioned substantial reductions in infections but resulted, for the first time, in a comprehensive description of chlamydia epidemiology. Although similar to gonorrhea in transmission and preferred tissue, it was shown to have a surprisingly dissimilar community form—a landmark epidemiologic observation, followed by a half dozen more. Our merging of contact tracing data with network analysis is shown to be one of the truly important analytic developments in STD/HIV epidemiology in the last half-century.

Five. Describes our 30-year public health association with prostitute women. Contact tracing led to sustained reductions in STD in prostitutes and to outstanding studies. We: showed that what makes a prostitute is likelier to be psychology than sociology; catalogued disorders associated with prostitution entry; suggested that psychological problems discourage prostitutes from using rehabilitative services; presented the first solid estimate of the number of prostitutes, and of career longevity in the US; provided the first (and only) study of mortality in prostitutes using the entire population; explained the nagging discrepancy in reported numbers of sexual partners by men and women; provided a valid estimate of prostitute clients in the US; an analysis of prostitution homicides and perpetrators; and quantified the deterrent effect on reoffending caused by police arrest of clients.

Six. Describes the first use of the network paradigm to assess the influence of network structure on transmission of infectious diseases. This study of prostitutes, injecting drug users, and their respective sexual and drug partners demonstrated that the social organization of relationships strongly influenced the magnitude and direction of HIV transmission. Changes in network conformation over time showed, for the first time, that the configuration of connections between people patterned HIV flow.

Seven. Critical examination of the view that sex is driving the HIV epidemics in Africa. Details the anomalies, dissonances, and stubborn facts that don't fit the official view of the international health agencies. Not only is the evidence they use anemic—studies do not control for confound between sexual and blood exposures—but it does not explain the turbocharged transmission observed, nor why "heterosexual transmission" is not sustained anywhere else in the world. Details the official resistance to conducting rigorous studies to settle the puzzle of HIV transmission in Africa. Distressingly, the official view is asserted with the arrogance of belief rather than with the humility of doubt.

Epilogue. Summarizes the geographic, bureaucratic, and operational contexts for our STD/HIV epidemiologic and control successes, emphasizing that low-tech interventions, enthusiasm for the work, tenacity, and luck were key ingredients.

Appendix one. Information Technology in our control endeavors.

Appendix two. Annotated list of our numerous scholarly letters to the editor.

Appendix three. Lists the numerous national, state, and local awards conferred.

Appendix four. Chronological list of conference presentations.

Appendix five. Timeline of overlapping control activities & formal studies.

PROLOGUE

For decades, *seeking the positive(s)* defined our award-winning sexually transmitted diseases control efforts, manner and matter. Manner, because the engine fueling them was enthusiasm for the work; matter, because their focus was on detecting positive cases, principally through contact tracing, our hallmark tactic. In brief, we sought the positive in both senses: the people who were unaware of being infected, and the optimism that powered our persistent efforts to find them.

While the high points of a career cannot be lived again, they can be remembered. Of concern is what is likelier to be remembered, fact or fiction. Memory is often faulty, not to mention selective, self-serving, and often embellished. Do we record what happened or what we like to think happened? Biographical story telling must be like science: rigorously self-critical. It must especially be mindful of the perils of self-sycophancy.

Mine was a long (nearly half a century) and rewarding career in public health. Or should I say "pubic health"? After all, it was devoted entirely to controlling sexually transmissible infections. Control was the principal aim—reducing the community burden of both bacterial and viral sexually transmissible infections. Yet, a funny thing happened along the way: the urgent need to figure out transmission dynamics in our own backyard. While the impact of our control initiatives was mostly confined to the Colorado Springs region, elucidation of local transmission dynamics had much broader applicability and reach. It turns out that in our particular experience was the universal. Hence this book, for this may be a story worth telling.

That these notable (as you shall soon see) contributions should have occurred under my watch as manager of a tiny sexually transmissible diseases control program in a small and obscure health department near the center of the continental United States is surprising and unexpected. Surprising and unexpected because of my unusual—if not eccentric—background. Equipped with only a bachelor's degree in medieval history (UCLA, '65) but also with a strong Protestant ethic, enthusiasm, and curiosity, this Swiss immigrant (1956, at age 14) found his public health calling quite by accident, shortly after the autumn of 1967, following a year's service with the 29th (Searchlight) Field Artillery in Vietnam's Central Highlands.

Despite my classical education in, and penchant for, the humanities I never neglected science or mathematics; indeed, starting in my early twenties, they became hobbies. Eric Burdon & The Animals once sang (in "Monterey", 1967): "You wanna find the truth in life, don't pass music by". Not only does this lyrical assertion accurately reflect the important role music (especially Rock 'n' Roll and Blues) has played in my life, but I can easily substitute the word "science" for "music" to describe its crucial influence in my personal and professional life. Science is how I know what I know, not religion or ideology. It's what has reliably guided me in the exploration of the usual questions: "How did we get here?"; "Why are we here?"; "What is the meaning of life?"; "Where is this all headed?" My intense personal, non-professional interest in science and mathematics spilled over into my calling: a lasting interest in infectious diseases and their expression in society. (My bedtime reading during my two-year stint in the Army usually consisted of books, such as those authored by Isaac Asimov, explaining science to a lay public. Physics and cosmology were particular favorites and have remained so to this day.)

"Autodidacts have the worst teachers"

—Woody Allen

Importantly, my weekly reading of medical, infectious disease, and public health journals while an employee of the health department allowed me to personally train and update my staff on relevant medical and epidemiologic topics via monthly meetings. This was of utmost importance, because there were seldom medical personnel or other educational resources available in our health department (or in our local hospitals) whose expertise in the medically unglamorous field of sexually transmissible agents was specialized enough to satisfy our needs, both as providers of STD services and as providers of accurate information to society at large. We had little choice but to rely on ourselves.

And now, the story.

ONE

ENHANCED CONTACT TRACING FOR STD/HIV:
OUR SECRET WEAPON

"The test of a vocation is the love of the drudgery it involves."

—L. P. Smith

Contact tracing: a tool to control the spread of
sexually transmissible diseases

The common thread that weaves through the fabric of my public health career is application of contact tracing to control STD/HIV epidemics. Contact tracing means actively seeking persons—"contacts"—who were exposed through sex, and (less often) through injecting drug use, with an infected person. The essential idea underlying this seemingly simple, if intrusive, act is to stop onward disease transmission—commonly referred to as "incidence". While it benefits individuals by alerting them to the possibility of being unknowingly infected, its real aim is to interrupt community-wide transmission. Contact tracing is much more about protecting populations than individuals, much more about protecting the uninfected than the infected.

Contact tracing has deep roots in public health practice. It likely originated to control venereal diseases in early 19th Century Europe, with Holland, Russia, and Sweden each being eligible for claiming pride of first place. But it wasn't until World War II that large-scale control programs were created in the United States, England, and Sweden.[1] Contact tracing was initially conceived as a tool to prevent spread. It was only later that other advantages were clearly recognized. Today, contact tracing is viewed as a control, epidemiologic, and ethical tool— an epidemiologic Swiss Army knife, if you will. Ethical, because it fulfills our moral duty to warn the unsuspecting; epidemiologic, because it provides on-the-ground evidence to elucidate transmission dynamics; and control, because it can interrupt onward transmission.

A brief overview might be useful. The fundamental tool of contact tracing is the contact interview, where the STD/HIV patient is asked to identify sexual contacts during a specified infectious period, and to provide locating information to ensure that exposed contacts will be notified, either by the patient (auto-referral) or health worker (contact tracing).[2] The latter is far more reliable than the former and, in the United States and Sweden, is used most often, especially for the serious STD. The notification process is completely confidential; the health worker never reveals the identity of the person who named them, nor any indirect information that might breach confidentiality. For example, the contact is never told the sex, occupation, residence, or locale/time of exposure, or the identity of the person who nominated him or her.

By the 1980s, the traditional view of contact tracing was changing. Opposition to it by gay activists early in the AIDS epidemic and the contemporaneous shift of public health orientation from the community to the individual was also mirrored in a nomenclature change, from *"contact tracing"* to *"partner notification"*.[3] The primary focus of contact tracing is on interrupting community transmission, while that of partner notification is on notifying one's contacts, whether done by public health workers or by the infected patient. The latter has a laissez-faire quality, while the former suggests snooping by a government agency. Viewing contact tracers as bedroom police is clearly a misperception, because the process of contact interviewing and contact tracing is *entirely* voluntary. Should a patient refuse to cooperate or choose to withhold information, there is nothing a public health worker could do other than try to make the patient see the importance of revealing relevant details. And while partner notification has its uses, it falls short of providing the full-bodied information needed to monitor and control STD epidemics. In short, partner notification is the shell of this public health intervention while contact tracing is its soul.[4] In Colorado Springs we did not waver in our commitment to contact tracing; if anything, we enhanced it. Not only did we conscientiously analyze routine contact tracing data but we enhanced the practice of contact tracing two ways: use of on-the-ground ethnographic observation and application of network analysis to collected data. (Ethnography describes the beliefs, customs, and behaviors of a group of people.)

"Never be afraid to try something new. Remember: amateurs built the Ark; professionals built the Titanic."

—Anonymous

Enter enhanced contact tracing

In its pro forma version, contact tracing simply consists of obtaining the names and locating information on contacts to infectious disease so that they can be referred to medical examination. End of story. *Enhanced* contact tracing is this basic process augmented by ethnography and by frequent data collation to discern connections between apparently unrelated transmission events. This is a thinking person's contact tracing endeavor. It provides the social context for transmission,[4] allowing you to see the forest for the trees. A graphic example serves to illustrate this process and its advantages. What follows outlines how enhanced contact tracing can fulfill its essential functions at once: ethical, epidemiologic, and control.

Chronicle of a gang-associated STD outbreak and its control

In the very early 1990s we successfully managed an intense outbreak of multiple STDs occurring in the social spaces of crack cocaine gangs. Their presence took us by complete surprise. As knowledgeable as we were with the presence and locations of populations at high risk for STD/HIV—having been boots-on-the-ground contact tracers for about a quarter century by then—we were unaware that crack cocaine gangsters from Los Angeles had arrived in Colorado Springs during 1988. Two rival gangs, the Crips and the Bloods, had formed in Los Angeles during the late 1960s. By the early 1980s their involvement in the crack cocaine trade had proved so lucrative that they expanded their markets elsewhere in America. This is what brought them to Colorado Springs. They first made their presence known to us via our VD Clinic in early 1990.

That year started with a bang. Two connected cases of penicillin-resistant gonorrhea (hereafter, PPNG) were diagnosed on the first working day of the year. This was highly unusual, because PPNG had only been sporadically diagnosed in Colorado since PPNG's near simultaneous discovery in East Asia and West Africa in 1976. The few cases that had been reported were usually diagnosed in military clinics, primarily among servicemen returning from East Asia; only 105 (0.5%) of the overall 19,726 gonorrhea cases recorded in Colorado Springs between 1976 and 1989 were PPNG cases.[5]

We did not recognize that these two January cases were part of a local PPNG outbreak until April, more than a hundred days later, by which time 6 total cases had been reported. And then all hell broke loose. What ensued was the most intense transmission of STD we witnessed during our four decades of STD control in Colorado Springs. The overall attack rate of more than 130,000 STD cases per 100,000 population that we witnessed during the 16-month period from December 1989—when the first case was retrospectively recognized—

and March 1991 represents, to my knowledge, the highest STD attack rate ever reported.[6]

Network analysis of the final contact tracing dataset comprised 410 sexually connected unique individuals, 218 men and 192 women, about 40% of whom had known gang affiliations; of the 410 people, 300 (about three-quarters) received medical examination. These 300 accounted for an astonishing 390 STD diagnoses (261 gonorrhea, 127 chlamydia, and 2 syphilis, cases). This undoubtedly represents a conservative tally for, given the relative insensitivity (40–60% accurate) of chlamydia tests used at the time, it is reasonable to suspect that at least an additional 100 diagnoses of chlamydia were missed. If so, then, the real attack rate exceeded 160,000 cases per 100,000 people. The 410 people in this gang-affiliated population represented a tiny 0.1 percent of the 18–44 year old population, yet accounted for 22 percent of all gonorrhea cases reported in Colorado Springs during that 16-month interval.

Natural partners: contact tracing and ethnography

It was one of our contact tracers, Perry Bethea who, by April 1990, first saw the forest for the trees: he recognized that the PPNG outbreak was occurring in the social spaces of street gangs associated with the crack cocaine trade. He had worked with street gangs the previous year in Denver, a city 65 miles north of Colorado Springs, and had acquired the confidence, vocabulary, and interest to work with them. He understood the distinction between alienated, which these people were, and aliens, which they were not. And although a long-haired 30-year old white male, he was able to gain the trust of gang members—principally African American men—and their ethnically diverse affiliates (young women and gang wannabes) who tended to be about ten years younger than he.

As detailed elsewhere,[6-7] Perry worked this outbreak on their turf—where gang members and their affiliates congregated: certain movie theaters, hamburger joints, shopping malls, public parks, and apartments. Apartments were key places because that was where sex and drug deals transpired. Being a constant presence in their social spaces made it easier to locate exposed contacts whose names and domiciles tended to be fluid. Street ethnography was a central feature of his interventions; it consists of two parts: see and be seen. Seeing things first hand helped him ask the right questions, while being seen promoted trust ("The temple of the familiar").

Network analysis (discussed in Chapter 6) of this outbreak revealed that 107 (of the 410 total gang members, affiliates, wannabes, and non-affiliates) people were densely connected sexually and responsible for the intensity of STD transmission. These 107 were more likely than the other 303 to be gang members rather than affiliates, to be very young, to have several STD diagnoses, and to name multiple sexual partners. Network analysis also provided strong support for the validity of ethnographic observations. For example, Perry was shown a names list of the 107 densely connected people and asked to select the 10 he would consider the most important actors in STD transmission during the outbreak; there was 70% concordance between Perry's picks and the network analysis computer program's picks. Notably, geographic mapping of the overall community's gonorrhea cases during this period, of the gang-associated cases, and of the PPNG cases revealed a fractal pattern—the best empiric demonstration of STD's fractal case distribution to date.[8] A fractal is a geometric pattern that repeats, but at different scales. In this instance, the geographic characteristics of gonorrhea were similar when viewed at the gang, neighborhood, or community-wide, case distribution scales.[8]

Lastly, Perry dealt with a brief recrudescence of gang-associated STD transmission, but it was short-lived (July–October 1991) and much less intense than the original outbreak. Knowledge distilled from field experience and social network analysis helped us intervene quickly and put out the transmission fires—something we had to do several times since, with similar happy results. Eternal vigilance comes with the STD control territory.

Conclusion and anticipation

In either of its two forms, simple or enhanced, contact tracing is straightforward in concept but difficult to successfully implement in reality. Obtaining the cooperation of members of the highest risk populations and finding the contacts they name—so many of whom have fluid lifestyles and impermanent addresses—takes imagination, optimism and, above all, tenacity. The importance of keeping good records and of periodically analyzing them for epidemiologic clues does not come naturally and takes considerable energy. One has to consciously plan, and make time, to achieve this goal.

In the United States, the Golden Age of contact tracing for STD unfolded during the three decades preceding 1980.[3] During this period there was little reason to explain or justify its practice to anyone, lay or professional; it was simply accepted as the right thing to do. The advent of intimidatingly large caseloads of bacterial STD, especially gonorrhea during the 1970s; of (re)nascent viral STD, especially genital herpes and AIDS in the 1980s; and of fierce opposition to its implementation by AIDS activists all contributed to devaluing contact tracing and to relegating it to the back seat, nay, the trunk of STD control engines. Our control program resolutely opposed these headwinds[3–4, 9] and not only continued to use contact tracing as its principal STD control engine, but found itself in position to educate segments of the public health establishment that did not clearly understand its safety, utility, efficacy, and effectiveness. Hence the long series of scholarly articles about contact tracing which started in 1984[10] and continued for thirty years.[11] Several textbook chapters detailed the history and track record of contact tracing,[3,10,12–13] while medical journal articles explained how contact tracing worked in real, as opposed to political or ideological, space.[2,4,14–15] We also strongly endorsed its use in HIV/AIDS control;[9,14,16] explained its utility and efficacy;[4,9,14] and advocated empirically-based improvements in contact tracing procedures.[17–19]

To summarize for the moment, and to anticipate our story: our many public health successes were the edifice that contact tracing built. It was conscientiously applied enhanced contact tracing that occasioned the frequent instances of incidence reductions recorded for gonorrhea, PPNG, chlamydia, and (to a lesser extent) HIV infections during our three decades of uninterrupted contact tracing in Colorado Springs; that elucidated the epidemiology and transmission dynamics of STD locally, but also had applicability for STD epidemiology in the rest of the world; that contributed substantially to elucidating the epidemiology of STD in pre-pubertal children; and that provided long-term data on the dynamics and perils of street prostitution.

As the following pages attest, we could not have made a better operational decision.

TWO

GONORRHEA CONTROL & EPIDEMIOLOGY

Before we get to the good parts, sketching some relevant background is necessary for framing how we got there.

Backstage: The late 1960s
(Enter John Potterat in Los Angeles County)

Each decade seems to "elect" its favorite venereal disease, to use an ancient and now abandoned term. When I started in the late 1960s, syphilis had the most "votes", as it had each decade since the beginning of that century. In the 1970s, gonorrhea replaced syphilis as best vote getter. In the 1980s, sexually transmissible viruses took pride of place—initially genital herpes and hepatitis-B but, most memorably, HIV/AIDS. During the 1990s, chlamydia and human papilloma virus ("venereal warts") emerged as favorites at the venereal "polls". Clearly, then, different sexually transmissible diseases (STD) play the role of squeaky hinge each decade and, therefore, get the most attention and lubricant (funding). But I'm getting ahead of the story, for this pattern was not generally recognized until roughly the mid-1970s.

1968 has been called the turning point year in the culture wars in the United States. Coincidentally, this story starts here—in early June when I first reported to work to begin my assignment for the Centers for

Disease Control's (CDC) Syphilis Eradication Program as a contact tracer assigned to the Los Angeles County Health Department. The office was a few blocks from the Ambassador Hotel where Robert Kennedy was shot shortly after midnight on June 5th. In those days, as now, people on the Right tended to view STD as a deserved consequence of immoral behavior, while those on the Left viewed it as a remediable public health problem. I was to spend 4 years as a contact tracer in various parts of Los Angeles County, initially in the black neighborhoods south of downtown, specifically Watts, a place where the vast majority of syphilis cases were diagnosed in young heterosexuals and, subsequently on the west side, specifically Hollywood, Beverly Hills, Santa Monica, Venice and Malibu, where the vast majority of cases were diagnosed in gay men. These were turbulent times. Civil rebellion ("Watts Riots") had erupted 3 years before, while the gay rebellion ("Stonewall Riots" in Manhattan's Greenwich Village, credited with triggering the "Gay Liberation" movement) was a year in the future.

These four years as a contact tracer in Los Angeles laid the groundwork not only for my STD control skills but, more importantly, for getting to know people from cultures very different from that of my white middle class background. In those early years, I saw mostly individual trees and only dimly perceived the forest patterns embedding them. As for people participating in STD transmission, I assumed that they were just like me, except that they happened to be gay, or black, or Hispanic, or hippies, or just unlucky. It took years of exposure to members of various populations to realize that differences were not superficial, but deeply cultural. I suppose that we are all inclined to assume that other people think just as we do, until we are shocked by some comment or observation into realizing that this is not necessarily so. Both the ability to see the forest for the trees of STD transmission, and the ability to understand that other people may view the world differently, turned out to be essential components of our eventual epidemiologic and control contributions. In brief: STD Basic Training took place in Los Angeles from 1968 to 1972, a few years after Army Basic Training at Fort Polk, Louisiana in the autumn of 1965.

Experiencing the San Fernando Valley earthquake in the early morning of 9 February 1971 convinced my family that moving to a more geologically stable place might be wise. One never knew when The Big One along the San Andreas Fault would occur, especially as the Los Angeles area kept experiencing aftershocks for nearly two weeks after the initial tremor. Eighteen months later we moved, without a job or job prospect, to a small community 1200 miles east, Colorado Springs, where my wife Susan had been a student at The Colorado College.

To anticipate: settling in Colorado Springs was the cornerstone blessing of my fortunate career, a land of STD epidemiologic opportunity— although this was not apparent at the time or, indeed, for years afterwards.

The Colorado Springs region, like the rest of America, was hosting a rapidly growing STD epidemic, especially gonorrhea, during the second half of the Sixties. Not only was this due to changing sexual mores associated with the hippie movement, and to the recent advent of an accurate diagnostic medium (Thayer-Martin culture for gonorrhea in 1964), but principally to Colorado Springs's huge military presence during the Vietnam War. In a small community (1970 census: 235,977) that had too few available women, the large numbers of young servicemen temporarily stationed locally (13% of total population), attracted itinerant camp followers and circuit prostitutes, many of whom were infected with gonorrhea and who, as we were soon to demonstrate, served as a continuous reservoir of infection.

During the late 1960s, the local health department had allocated only modest resources to controlling STD; their VD Clinic (as it was called in the old days) offered services only a few hours a week, and only one employee was given the duty of tracing infections in the community, almost exclusively gonorrhea. (Tracing contacts to the "really important" STD, syphilis, was tasked to CDC's Syphilis Control Program assignee based in Denver, 65 miles due north.) By 1970, the health department could no longer ignore the rapid rise in reported gonorrhea cases and the stage was set for motivated, energetic individuals to capitalize on this public health opportunity: combating a newly renascent and rapidly spreading STD in a community with little epidemiologic or bureaucratic STD control experience. Unlike syphilis, which not only occurred much less frequently than gonorrhea, but had a public health control tradition dating to at least the late 1930s, gonorrhea control had received only modest attention nationally since World War II. In short, the gonorrhea stage was unfettered by bureaucratic precedent, either national or local. A control program could select its own actors and write its own script. Hence the opportunity to experiment with control measures rather than following a prescribed, predigested protocol, as was the case with the CDC's national syphilis control endeavor, which was highly choreographed. To paraphrase Tip O'Neill, "All gonorrhea control is local".[1]

Backstage: The early 1970s in Colorado Springs sans John Potterat

The principal reason for controlling gonorrhea, a relatively mild disease, was to prevent reproductive tract damage, especially infertility in young women. And the motivated, energetic individual who got the ball rolling was the health department's newly appointed director in February of 1970, Dr. Hugh H. Rohrer, who marshaled the community's resources—medical, political, legal, and military—to counter the gonorrhea tide. And a rapidly rising tide it was, with reported cases having dramatically increased from 408 in 1964 to 663 in 1968 to 1,659 in 1970. Ethnographic studies, courtesy of the American Social Health Association, and interviewing of infected patients, indicated that the vast majority of gonorrhea cases occurred in young servicemen providing a history of recent sexual contact with a prostitute or camp follower. As we detailed elsewhere[2] and partially quote here:

Initial control efforts mobilized public health workers, criminal justice officials, and the media. Briefly, civilian and military health workers interviewed STI patients and attempted field follow-up of named partners. Military policemen enforced proscription directed at interdicted sites frequented by soldiers suspected of soliciting commercial sex. Civilian police enhanced their efforts to repress prostitution by creating a special monitoring unit, the vice-squad. The District Attorney [Bob Russel] pressed for vigorous prosecution and for creative sentencing of persons engaging in prostitution. (For example, "hiccup" sentences were imposed on persons convicted of prostitution: instead of imposing a continuous 90-day sentence, judges meted out sentences that confined the prisoner to jail from the 25th day of a month to the 5th day of the next. Generally, this occurred over a three-month period; its purpose was to discourage prostitution on or about military payday.) The media alerted the public to the burgeoning gonorrhea epidemic and encouraged residents to consider legalizing prostitution in this military environment. Two additional observations deeply influenced the decision to invoke the public health authority during the emerging gonorrhea epidemic: the peripatetic lifestyle of most women engaging in prostitution locally and their apparently cavalier attitude toward venereal infection. First, ethnographic data suggested that more than half of prostitutes followed a professional circuit that comprised several neighboring states; these women solicited clients locally for the few days surrounding military payday and then resumed travel on the circuit. Estimates based on sporadic medical examination and on contact tracing information suggested that at least one third of such women had sexually transmissible infections and that most eluded public health interventions in other communities within their circuit. Second, conventional STI control measures (e.g., contact tracing and street outreach) were failing to successfully refer prostitutes to medical care: a fluid lifestyle without permanent domicile, a rather fatalistic and stoical approach to life's problems, and a major concern with sheer survival served to relegate the seeking of health care to a low priority. Accordingly, a legal system requiring public health clearance of persons arrested for prostitution offenses, the "Health Hold Order", was initiated by the health department in Colorado Springs in June, 1970. In practice, a person arrested for prostitution was permitted to post bond only after a health department representative made a determination of the likelihood that the detainee had an STI. Such determination was made either directly (that is, based on results of standard gonorrhea cultures and syphilis serologies obtained by the health department or by a licensed local clinician in the 30 days preceding arrest) or indirectly (based on results of such tests collected from the population of prostitutes tested locally). Using a standard of "reasonable suspicion" (being suspected of engaging in prostitution locally and therefore of likelihood of having a reportable STI), such persons were detained for a period not exceeding 72 hours to permit examination by a qualified practitioner. Persons arrested for prostitution were examined and treated at our health department STI clinic free of charge; those for whom reasonable suspicion was absent were permitted to post bond immediately."

Another energetic and motivated individual, Mark Brecher, was hired to manage the VD Clinic and control program. A reluctantly transplanted New Yorker who arrived in Colorado Springs because his wife was stationed at Fort Carson as an Army nurse, Mark nevertheless threw himself into the task, all cylinders firing. With no background in medicine or public health other than a two-week formal CDC course on STD contact interviewing and contact tracing, he laid the foundation for active STD case reporting, comprehensive prostitution surveillance, gonorrhea case-finding via contact tracing, not to mention the critical component of establishing a close working relationship with local military public health authorities. By the summer of 1972, after

21

about 2 years of single-handedly running the STD control program for the local health department, he realized that without additional help much would remain undone, especially contact tracing, which presently took a backseat to implementation of a new federal gonorrhea screening program. This program, initially funded for fiscal year 1972, required visiting local physicians in medical practices, both private and quasi-private (Planned Parenthood and Free clinics), likely to be assessing patients for genitourinary, birth control, or pregnancy related, conditions. It had been made possible by the development of a transportable version of the Thayer-Martin culture medium ("Transgrow"), which consisted of a little glass bottle lined with the medium and sealed with the gas that gonorrhea bacteria needed to grow: carbon dioxide. A courier service collected Transgrow specimens obtained by private practitioners 5 days a week for delivery to the health department laboratory, which tested the specimens free of charge. Persuading each physician to screen susceptible patients took months of personal visits by Mark, who relied on his considerable charm and, above all, dogged persistence to get the job done.

Front-stage: The early 1970s
(enter John Potterat in Colorado Springs)

Because it was thought that the private sector gonorrhea screening program was likely to function on automatic pilot after the initial time investment of personal visits to physicians, Mark requested temporary help only. This is how and where I came in. By chance and, it turns out, fantastic luck, I was to become the temporary hire. How? A health department nurse happened to be my neighbor and, after inquiring about my professional background, mentioned that Mark was looking for short-term help, and that my qualifications might well fit the requirements. After a brief interview, Mark offered me a 90-day contract, paid via the Colorado State Department of Health's STD control budget, to perform STD contact tracing—especially syphilis contact tracing, since the Colorado Springs region was experiencing a sudden surge in infectious cases. He apologized that he could not offer a salary approaching what I had been paid by the CDC for the same work. I accepted anyway. Start date? Monday 2 October 1972, a short 36 days after our arriving and settling in Colorado Springs without a job.

Mark and I worked beautifully together. We were both young, idealistic, and dedicated. His two-year front lines apprenticeship in gonorrhea control and street ethnography, particularly with street prostitutes, blended well with my Los Angeles apprenticeship in syphilis control and street ethnography in Hollywood's gay cruising locales. He frequented the street and bar venues hosting pimps and prostitutes, and I frequented Colorado Springs's gay venues—although we each cross-visited each of these epidemiologically important STD loci. Just before termination of my 90-day contract, Mark asked the State Health Department for a six-month extension, a request granted by the Colorado State Epidemiologist, Dr. Thomas M. Vernon. Mark was planning on returning to New York upon termination of his wife's

23

Army obligation at the end of June 1973, and was thus grooming me to take over his excellent program, contingent on approval by the VD Program's supervisor, the Director of the Nursing Division, Frieda Laubach.

Frieda consented, and I was assigned to run both the VD clinic and control program as a full time employee of the El Paso County (hereafter: Colorado Springs) Health Department, starting 1 July 1973. Needless to say, these two tasks exceeded one person's ability to do them justice, especially during the year's busiest time. Gonorrhea was a disease of pronounced seasonality, with substantial increases in reported cases occurring during the year's third quarter. A hectic summer—not to mention that my wife was pregnant with our first child—helped persuade Frieda that help was needed. Since local funding for such a position was not likely to be found, an appeal was made to the Colorado Department of Health in Denver which, because it received funding to control STD directly from the CDC, agreed to create a position in its VD Control Program, assigning a State employee to Colorado Springs.

This noble act was not a disinterested one, for the State Health Department likely wanted greater control over the traditionally independent Colorado Springs program. Indeed, this was the only VD program in Colorado not directly controlled by state health authorities. This independence was a consequence of the United States Army situating Camp Carson about a dozen miles south of Colorado Springs in 1942. The sudden infusion of about 20,000 young men in a community of, at the time, only about 40,000 people stimulated the arrival of female camp followers and, unsurprisingly, of venereal diseases. The local health department and military authorities cooperated in combating VD, mostly independently of the distant Colorado Department of Health in Denver. By 1973, Colorado Springs had dealt with the sudden infusion of large numbers of servicemen and venereal diseases during 4 wars: World War II, the Korean War, the Cold War, and the Vietnam War. These continuous and largely contiguous occurrences helped consolidate the tradition of independent local VD control efforts. Although Mark had had a very good relationship with the State Health Department VD control staff, he cherished and maintained this traditional independence, and its freedom from deadening and potentially obstructionist bureaucratic overlays. I was philosophically and psychologically in sync, for independence suited my intellectual and personality inclinations.

Front stage: Enter Christopher I. Pratts and Lynanne Phillips, STD superstars

The person who won the Colorado State Health Department competition to fill the Colorado Springs position was Chris Pratts; he received the highest score on the entrance examination. He was to serve as principal STD contact tracer for more than twenty years, starting in October 1973. At about the same time I, who had served as a part-time Contact Interviewing School instructor for the CDC during the very early 1970s, began to formally train the health department nurses who were periodically assigned to staff VD Clinic by the Nursing Division. One, Lynanne Phillips RN, who volunteered to work the afterhours VD clinic, proved exceptionally gifted at interviewing and counseling patients. Like Chris Pratts, Lynanne was very bright, intuitive, empathetic, curious, and highly motivated.

The 1970s: The Gonorrhea Decade
(Enter the CDC's Richard Rothenberg, MD MPH)

The VD Program now had sufficient resources to at least maintain, though preferably improve upon, the successes achieved during Mark's tenure. Of greater significance for the long run was my fortuitous introduction to Dr. Richard Rothenberg at a Colorado State VD Program meeting in Vail in October 1974. The CDC's concern for the rapidly expanding gonorrhea epidemic, which was soon to reach one million reported cases annually in the United States, generated the pressing need to better understand both gonorrhea's transmission dynamics on the community level and fertility-threatening tissue damage, especially in young women. Consequently, the CDC assigned the young Dr. Jim Curran to Columbus, Ohio, and the equally young Dr. Rothenberg to Denver, Colorado, "to support the establishment of comprehensive data systems and to monitor the impact of current programmes" [3] —young doctors for a young person's disease, a consonant choice. Incidentally, Dr. Curran was to achieve fame 7 years later as the head of the task force for the newly identified infectious disease GRID [Gay Related Immune Deficiency], later renamed HIV/AIDS.

I initially met not Dr. Rothenberg, but his gregarious wife Carol (present with their 8 month-old son Leon), with whom I talked about a mutual interest: Hi-Fi stereo equipment. Only shortly after did I meet her seemingly introverted, brilliant husband. Dr. Rothenberg explained what his CDC mission and interests were while I, in turn, provided brief details of our gonorrhea control endeavors in Colorado Springs, including our unconventional use of the Health Hold Order to control the flow of gonorrhea from itinerant street prostitutes.

Our First Formal Study

In 1974 we only had adequate resources to interview men with urethral gonorrhea, to assure treatment of their usually silently infected female contacts. Indeed, this was the approach recommended by the CDC. The other side of the coin, the interviewing of women with gonorrhea to assure treatment of their male sexual contacts was thought to be unnecessary, because it was assumed that infected men would have external symptoms. At about that time, one of us (Lynanne Phillips) began to suspect that, by not interviewing women with gonorrhea, we might be losing an opportunity to refer those among their sexual contacts who had no urethral symptoms, or who were insufficiently inconvenienced by mild symptoms, to seek medical care. Because the procedure was not recommended by the CDC; because we did not have adequate resources to interview infected women and to trace their contacts; and because we were unaware of any program data showing its utility, the only way we could pursue this epidemiologic insight was to interview fewer men or/and place these men on an honor system: "Please inform your contacts yourself and refer them to a clinic".

This "self-referral" approach for men with gonorrhea had recently been tried on a pilot basis in Baltimore[4]—subsequently receiving a CDC young investigator award—but not reported in the public health literature. Being a trained epidemiologic investigator, and recognizing the potential importance of doing such a study rigorously so that it could appear in a scholarly journal, Dr. Rothenberg suggested that we structure a formal investigation, complete with study (self-referral method) and control (formal health department contact tracing) groups. It began in February 1975, a few months after we initially met. He was the study's principal architect and formal scientific mentor, for none of us in the Colorado Springs program had had any exposure to either structuring or reporting studies for biomedical journals. Indeed, it had never even crossed our minds that we, none of whom had advanced degrees or training, should or could do this. It was to become our first published paper,[5] empirically demonstrating that the female contacts to men with gonorrhea were equally likely to be successfully referred to medical care via the self-referral or the formal contact tracing routes. Dr. Rothenberg's initial advice: "As long as you're going to be trying this, why don't you do it formally?" could be called his modus operandi, if not his motto; it was to influence virtually all subsequent VD empiric studies in Colorado Springs.

The 1970s: Our Three Notable Accomplishments
in Gonorrhea Epidemiology

The principal strength of our program has been the willingness and ability to do meticulous field follow-up of STD cases and to maintain complete records. This enabled us to collect and analyze quality empiric data, which were used not only to monitor our progress in STD control but to justify our often unconventional, if not controversial, interventions. The notable early accomplishments in our gonorrhea control efforts during the 1970s were to 1) detail the importance of actively identifying and treating non-symptomatic male gonorrhea carriers, 2) demonstrate that community transmission could be controlled, even in the absence of a vaccine, and 3) provide detailed evidence to support Yorke and colleagues' Core Group Theory.[6]

In the mid-1970s, Dr. Rothenberg's special interest was Core Group Theory, the recent brainchild of a CDC funded mathematical modeling endeavor.[6] Rothenberg was a gifted abstract and quantitative thinker; hence the theory, which was developed by a group of researchers headed by James A. Yorke[6] (later of Chaos Theory fame), appealed to him because of its conceptual framing and mathematical rigor. In brief, the theory postulates that only a small proportion of gonorrhea patients, directly or indirectly, contribute most of the gonorrhea transmission in the community and that, by extension, if these successful transmitters could have their infection intercepted by public health interventions, then removal of their infection from the disease pool would have disproportionate impact on gonorrhea incidence. Huge bang for small bucks, as it were. Dr. Rothenberg went fishing for empiric evidence for this appealing and promising theory. He found it in Colorado Springs.

Using the specially flagged VD Clinic medical charts of prostitute women, and the separate logbooks used to monitor the frequency of their visits under the Health Hold Order system, Dr. Rothenberg was able to provide initial empiric support for the Core Group concept by showing that, likelier than not, about one-third of all gonorrhea cases in Colorado Springs could be attributed to about 3% of the infected population, in this case, street prostitutes.[7] But it was likely that there would be other core groups as well.

Pleased with the quality of the available VD Program data in Colorado Springs and with the competence and enthusiasm of its contact tracing staff, Dr. Rothenberg successfully sought funding from his parent agency, the CDC, to conduct a focused study to identify categories of core group transmitters other than street prostitutes. With this CDC funding, Lynanne Phillips, a public health nurse who had been working part-time in VD Clinic during the preceding 4 years, was hired full-time in 1976 to empirically test the nagging suspicion that certain categories of women with gonorrhea might be contributing disproportionately to gonorrhea transmission. Such women seemingly shared one attribute: the circumstances surrounding their diagnosis *implied* the presence of non-symptomatic infected males in their sexual environments. These non-symptomatic male carriers could be found principally in 3 categories of female cases: women with gonococcal pelvic inflammatory disease; women whose diagnosis was a consequence of screening for infection; and women with a repeat episode within a few months of their original infection. In each case, it could be inferred that had these women's sexual contacts been symptomatic (frank urethral discharge and/or burning), their contacts would have sought treatment; instead, these men were probably minimally or non-symptomatic, remaining silently infected and infectious long enough to unsuspectingly contribute many cases downstream. We viewed them as the likeliest substrate for the stubborn entrenchment of gonorrhea in the community.

> "The one who says it cannot be done should never interrupt the one who is doing it."
>
> —The Roman Rule

Contact tracing's gift to gonorrhea control: They said it couldn't be done

Not only was Lynanne's epidemiologic insight confirmed (three-fifths of infected contacts to these women were shown to be minimally- or non-symptomatic[8-10]), but assiduous tracing and treating of these silently infected men was associated with a substantial decline in gonorrhea cases.[8,10] This empiric evidence countered the prevailing view that doubted, if not the existence of non-symptomatic male carriers, at least their importance in sustaining gonorrhea transmission. The tacit understanding that gonorrhea was a self-limited disease in men promoted this misconception. (Self-limited means that, with time, the infection would go away by itself.) Importantly, this pioneering study also provided strong support for the hypothesis advanced by Core Group theorists that concentrating on a small proportion of infected cases could have a disproportionate impact on the community gonorrhea burden; in this case, contact tracing efforts which focused on treating the silently infected male contacts of fewer than 30% of specially designated women (those in the 3 categories in the above paragraph), who represented only 10% of all (male and female) cases, was associated with a 23% decline in gonorrhea cases during the 2-year study interval, not to mention a 35% decline in cases of pelvic inflammatory disease (PID)—the most common serious complication of gonococcal infection in women.[11] These were welcome results, for they countered the prevailing pessimistic view in public health circles that gonorrhea transmission occurred too rapidly and that there were, in any event, far too many cases to interview, to hope for community gonorrhea control and for reduction in complications (like PID) in the absence of a vaccine.

Targeted gonorrhea control efforts during the second half of the 1970s in Colorado Springs, which concentrated intervention energies in small, definable core groups, constituted the first prospectively documented empiric demonstration that focal use of contact tracing could substantially diminish gonorrhea incidence. Contemporaneous use of conventional (non-focal) contact tracing had been associated with similar incidence reductions in Sheffield and Newcastle, England, both of which health districts had used contact tracing to control gonorrhea since World War II[12–13] but their data were insufficiently complete to convince doubters. That our meticulously documented and nearly complete observations were important is attested by the fact that they were published in major biomedical journals, including the *American Journal of Public Health*[8], the *American Journal of Obstetrics and Gynecology*[9] and, especially, the *Journal of the American Medical Association*[10], which not only placed this latter as their weekly issue's lead article, but also editorialized it.[14]

To our surprise, these encouraging observations and allied recommendations were not programmatically advocated by either Federal or State (including Colorado!) gonorrhea control organizations. Not only had the public health establishment averred that it couldn't be done, but its subsequent programmatic silence showed that, should it be done, it could be rationalized away or simply ignored. After all, in their view, this was Colorado Springs and Colorado Springs was a special case: its results did not really apply elsewhere, not even elsewhere in Colorado! (It was Dr. Rothenberg who later quipped that I "was a prophet without honor in his own country".) Regrettably, as we shall see, this was not to be the last ironic conclusion to be drawn

33

from our sexually transmitted diseases control efforts or innovations
—past, present, or future.

Second time a charm?
(Enter Donald E. Woodhouse, budding STD Superstar)

Conscientious use of contact tracing to further reduce gonorrhea
incidence in Colorado Springs was implemented in the late 1970s.
During the preceding few years, it had become painfully clear that the
military presence (about 30,000 uniformed personnel out of the 1980
Census population of 309,424) was currently contributing most of the
remaining gonorrhea burden now that civilian cases and cases among
street prostitutes had substantially declined. Worse, the military
personnel tasked with interviewing infected patients in their own
medical venues were poorly motivated to perform quality contact
interviewing and tracing. As Colorado Springs VD control program
director, I pleaded this case to military public health authorities, using
hard data from the previous 3 years, to get permission to assign and,
equally importantly, to fund one civilian VD contact tracer in Fort
Carson's infectious diseases unit. Pressure from an influential
community member on our Board of Health helped persuade initially
reluctant military authorities to authorize and fund the requested
position. It was quickly filled by newcomer Donald Woodhouse, an
enthusiastic if yet untrained contact tracer. As detailed in the journal
Public Health Reports, [15] Woodhouse transformed the culture of VD
control mediocrity at Fort Carson to one of exceptional contact tracing

outcomes. Indeed, his impressive performance convinced the military to continue funding this civilian position after his departure in 1982 (when he left to attend law school in Denver) for the next quarter century.

Pointing the finger at deficiencies in the Army Post's infectious diseases unit was accompanied by self finger-pointing at our own VD program's weaknesses: only half of gonorrhea cases diagnosed in the civilian sector were routinely interviewed for contact information—those in public or quasi-public clinics. Indeed, most cases diagnosed in private doctors' offices and in hospital emergency rooms had never been routinely sought out for contact tracing purposes. Starting in late 1979, saturation contact tracing was implemented to gauge the magnitude of its impact on local incidence: >90% of all reported gonorrhea cases from all medical venues, civilian and military, were interviewed and their contacts actively sought for treatment. By the end of 1982, community gonorrhea cases had declined a further 17%. In both instances (1976–1978 and 1980–1982) the distribution of cases and their diagnostic categories changed substantially in ways that provided exceptional evidence that the noted incidence reductions were likely caused by the specific contact tracing initiatives implemented.[8,10,15] In brief we had substantially changed the complexion of our community's gonorrhea cases, from diagnostic categories largely reflecting downstream (passive), to those suggesting upstream (active), detection. In the mid-1970s, the director of the national VD control program at the CDC, Dr. Ralph H. Henderson, had referred to contact tracing as the "sleeping giant" of VD control. Ironically, empirically demonstrating the wisdom of his remark with high quality evidence, on two separate occasions in a period of six years, apparently failed to sufficiently impress his successors at the CDC and the rest of the public health establishment, for no recommendation to broaden focal use of gonorrhea contact tracing to identify and treat male carriers was advocated. In short, the second time was not a charm, any more than the first.

Gonorrhea in pre-pubertal children: An illuminating tangent

Use of contact tracing and the importance of non-symptomatic infection also played an important role in the elucidation of gonorrhea transmission not simply in Colorado Springs adults, but in several of its infected children. Although neither our local nor State health department had any known previous experience with the epidemiology of gonorrhea infection in young children—a reportedly rare occurrence—I decided to follow-up on case reports. During the thirteen months separating July 1975 and August 1976, several pre-pubertal cases were reported from local hospital emergency rooms. As detailed in our second publication, [16] each case was carefully investigated. An important epidemiologic pattern emerged: in each household hosting an infected pre-pubertal girl, an adult woman with gonorrhea reported contact with an adult man (boyfriend or other man) who denied symptoms and who, when subsequently referred to examination, was shown to be infected. In each instance, the infected carrier denied sexual contact with the child, although each had had opportunity to be alone with the infected child. We persistently and firmly pressured all adults and all other children in these households to be tested for gonorrhea. This meticulous investigation also yielded the first reported case in the literature of non-symptomatic infection in a pre-pubertal girl: a 2-year old had positive gonorrhea cultures from the urethra, vagina, and anus in the absence of symptoms.[16] These baptism-under-fire investigations gave us the experience and confidence for the proper management of subsequent cases, however infrequently these were occurring.

Especially notable was an equally meticulous investigation, conducted ten years later, of 3 related gonorrhea cases in children residing in a trailer park. Although the pattern among the adults was similar (women with gonorrhea whose infected male partners were non-symptomatic), the important observation was that contact tracing identified a pre-pubertal boy with non-symptomatic urethral gonorrhea. Even more remarkably, this 7-year-old boy admitted in graphic detail to having been seduced by a 5-year-old infected neighbor girl ("She told me she knew how to make it hard and what to do with it"), the same girl who had infected the 4-year-old index case. This report can be viewed as the first well-documented case of child-to-child gonorrhea transmission in the literature.[17] And the tenacious health department nurse who persisted long enough to elicit this stunningly descriptive statement was the grandmotherly and angelically patient Helen P. Zimmerman, RN. An interviewing tour de force indeed!

Elucidating gonorrhea transmission dynamics

Gonorrhea's renaissance during the 1960s was unexpected. Following routine use of penicillin during the second half of the 1940s, gonorrhea incidence had dramatically declined, reaching a nadir in reported cases by 1957. But evidence that it might be on the rebound emerged by the early 1960s. Nationally, reported cases more than tripled, from 300,666 in 1964 to 1,001,994 by 1976, the peak year for this surprisingly rapid epidemic. (Part of the dramatic increase can be attributed to introduction of a much improved diagnostic test in 1964.) At the time, many authorities believed that the best chance to control gonorrhea lay with a vaccine rather than through contact tracing. Contact tracing was seriously advocated and used to control infectious syphilis, a venereal disease that, because it had a long and non-infectious incubation period (10–90 days), afforded public health workers sufficient time to head the disease off at the pass, meaning to treat exposed contacts before the end of their incubation period. In addition, its moderate transmission efficiency made syphilis a manageable public health problem; its transmission attributes were inherently considerably slower than those of gonorrhea. Not only did gonorrhea lack a non-infectious incubation period, but its transmission efficiency was high: about 50% per unprotected sexual exposure for the woman and about 20% for the man, not to mention much higher if the woman was using birth control pills. Such data suggested that interrupting gonorrhea transmission using contact tracing was a Sisyphean task—endless and ineffective— because efficient transmission was bound to outrun public health

38

interventions. Other than educating the public, screening for non-symptomatic infection in young women undergoing a pelvic examination was regarded as the most promising intervention. Because men were thought to almost always show symptoms, the provision of free clinics to treat them and their partners was considered sufficient;[3] hence gonorrhea contact tracing services were only recommended for symptomatic men because, like the screening program, they would point to untreated, infected women.

The rapid transmission of gonorrhea in many American communities from the mid-1960s through the 1970s also helped foster the view that, if you were young and sexually non-monogamous, you were at risk of acquiring it. This democratic view ("anyone can get it") of gonorrhea, though useful for obtaining public funding for its control, did not reflect reality on the ground.

I must admit that even I, who began interviewing gonorrhea patients in the autumn of 1972, uncritically believed that this view was correct. My training in syphilis contact tracing had introduced me to patients (older, browner, and often gay) who were very different from those I now interviewed for gonorrhea (young, white, and heterosexual). The reality was that, over time, our gonorrhea contact tracing efforts frequently took us to the same few neighborhoods, the same few taverns, the same streets, and even the same addresses, now with different occupants. This observation could have been made by anyone doing contact tracing in any American community large enough to sustain its own transmission chains, especially if the contact tracer remained on duty long enough before being transferred to another jurisdiction or before leaving the profession. In our case, it took about two years to notice this pattern and a few more to realize that such a pattern may not be due to chance.

The importance of working in VD Clinic,
rather than being a peripheral health worker

During the same period, our contact tracers were also assigned to conduct initial medical intake on any patient attending our VD Clinic. This was unusual, because contact tracers were narrowly tasked only with interviewing positive cases and assuring treatment for their contacts. This was because such duties left little time for the less difficult and admittedly less time-consuming task of recording basic medical information in VD Clinic, something usually completed by lower level medical personnel. That our contact tracers were also expected to conduct medical intake on any patient during clinic hours exposed them to the world of patients without gonorrhea or syphilis, like the worried well or patients with minor genital or urinary tract conditions. This was, in effect, a natural control group. In retrospect this was a fortunate decision, initially made by Mark Brecher, for it helped merge two different VD perspectives: the clinical and the epidemiologic. Most contact tracers in the United States worked within a specialized job description and were under-exposed to the world of clinical medicine.

This dual exposure in our VD Clinic is what eventually led to my first epiphany: that sex alone could not be the crucial risk factor for gonorrhea. Although it took a long time for this realization to find clear form, what I was beginning to see was that sex was a necessary, but not sufficient, cause for acquiring the disease. Nor could infection be attributed to bad luck. Although this realization also took time to coalesce in my mind, it occurred to me that visiting the same bars, the same addresses, the same neighborhoods over and over again, suggested that there was a connection between risk of infection and these facts. What most influenced my thinking was confronting the uncomfortable fact that life was not fair: in talking to so many different patients in VD Clinic, some of whom were not infected with gonorrhea despite their adventurous sexual lives and, at the other end of the spectrum, talking with a few who frequently acquired gonorrhea even though they revealed conservative sexual lives, I soon became convinced that gonorrhea risk could not be as randomly or evenly distributed as routine health education messages were advertising. Especially important was frequent observation of this dissonance. And especially striking was the difference in gonorrhea test outcome between sexually adventurous white women from a local upper middle class college and similarly aged black women with modest sexual histories and educational backgrounds. The former were seldom diagnosed with gonorrhea, unlike the latter. This recurring observation not only offended my innate sense of justice but, more importantly, piqued my curiosity. I needed to know why. However, we were so intent on our principal task, reducing the community burden of gonorrhea, and so busy with large caseloads and paperwork duties that curiosity took a back seat to quotidian duties.

Contact tracing's gift to VD epidemiology:
Gonorrhea as a social disease

As Dr. Rothenberg was fond of pointing out, contact tracing's strength is that it takes you where the problem is. By problem, he meant as close to disease transmission events as possible. Since our principal concern was to substantially interrupt gonorrhea transmission in Colorado Springs, we needed to delineate the most intense transmission milieux; we could then concentrate intervention energies to the hot spots, hoping, nay trusting, that this rifling approach would have disproportionate impact on community transmission, as predicted by Core Group Theory. Implementation of saturation contact tracing in late 1979 can be viewed as equivalent to sustained, relentless frontal attacks by boots on the ground, in this case contact tracers in the field. Although our primary aim was rapid incidence reduction, an important secondary aim of saturation contact tracing was to develop a sense for under-reporting of gonorrhea cases in the private medical sector, because one of the criticisms of our first gonorrhea incidence reduction success was that we were not seeing unreported cases, especially those treated in private doctors' offices; hence our claims of success were probably premature.

Our team, especially Don Woodhouse and I, spent many hours reflecting on the data being collected during the first year of saturation contact tracing (calendar 1980). They not only provided convincing evidence that unreported gonorrhea cases were a rarity in Colorado Springs but, far more importantly, they pointed to the need to collect additional information. In manually (we had no computers) linking patients and their contacts, clustering patterns emerged. These were noted because we had decided to pool cases and contacts in so-called lots. The lot system had been developed at the CDC many years before to connect syphilis cases;[3] we applied it to gonorrhea. Woodhouse spent much time examining highly connected lots, hand plotting case-contact pairs on a time continuum (Scotch-taping legal-pad sized sheets!). From these primitive graphs emerged a fairly clear picture of who the intense transmission actors were in 1980, along with a better sense for how far behind the epidemiologic events our current contact tracing efforts were. It was only many years later that it dawned on us that lot system analysis and graphing of connections was really an unconscious use of network analysis (see Chapter 6).

In addition, because Woodhouse and I spent many hours in the field, we became more familiar than previously with the places where high-risk patients socialized. Such observations led us to embed a special study in context of saturation contact tracing. Sometime in the autumn of 1980 we decided to add several questions to the standard contact interview, questions intended to place the individual and her contacts in a social context. For example, gonorrhea patients were now routinely asked not simply for the names, sexual exposure information and locating details of their contacts, but also how long they had lived at their present address; how long they had known their sexual contact before first having sex with them; where they had met; and where they liked to socialize. This embedded study was intended to span calendar year 1981, but was terminated midway because we were not able to obtain additional funding to assure uninterrupted saturation interviewing, especially during the summer months when our staff customarily took annual leave. In short, we ran out of gas, although we continued intensive contact tracing, but without obtaining the additional, social information. It turns out that these few additional questions, embedded in an endeavor aimed principally at reducing gonorrhea incidence, yielded a picture much more important than the sum of its parts. Indeed, it led to publication of our first landmark paper several years later, "Gonorrhea as a social disease".[18]

The popular view had been that gonorrhea patients could come from any part of the community but were, like many young people, impulsive, peripatetic, and socially unstable. From our embedded study data emerged a strikingly different picture, one of highly focal concentration: demographically, ethnically, socially, residentially, and geographically. Indeed, they provided the first incontrovertible evidence for Core Group Theory's validity—the theory which posited that small, definable, stable, sexually active groups were responsible for maintaining gonorrhea in the community through intragroup sexual contacts. Our data fit the theory like a glove. These showed that half of all gonorrhea cases occurred in people living in a mere 4 (6%) of the 68 census tracts in Colorado Springs and that the addition of 9 census tracts accounted for three-quarters of all cases; the same was true for their contacts, as sexual partner choices were socio-geographically homophilous (like chooses like). As for socialization, 6 establishments (2% of all those mentioned by patients) accounted for half of all citations of sites of social aggregation by gonorrhea patients. Demographically, gonorrhea cases were concentrated in only 1% of people aged 15 to 34 years, and were also highly concentrated in non-white heterosexuals of lower socioeconomic extraction, and connected to the military. Cases exhibited not only residential proximity but, surprisingly, residential stability, with nearly half of cases having not moved in at least six months and nearly 40% having lived at their address more than one year. As for the period of social acquaintanceship preceding the first sexual liaison, 45% of case-contact pairs had known each other for more than two months, and 18% more than a year, prior to first sex. So much for the democratic "everyone is at risk" message; so much for the randomly-evenly distributed view; and so much for the "impulsive, peripatetic, socially unstable" parts. Gonorrhea was truly a social disease, with risk of disease acquisition firmly entrenched in socio-geographic space ("Potterat structures"[19–20]). And yes, "social disease" was inspired by "*West Side Story*", a favorite film for both Dr. Rothenberg and me.

Mining this nearly complete data set for
additional useful epidemiologic information

After 5 years in Colorado Dr. Rothenberg was, to both our chagrin and selfish concern, reassigned by the CDC to the State health department in Albany, New York; this was also the year that his boss, Dr. Ralph Henderson, accepted assignment to the World Health Organization in Geneva. Thus, these departures preceded implementation of our saturation contact tracing campaign in late 1979. We were especially concerned about prospectively losing Dr. Rothenberg's analytic skills, not to mention that he had access to, and knew how to program, mainframe computers and was conversant in advanced statistical analysis programs. No one at the Colorado Springs health department had either computers or data-exploratory expertise beyond simple analyses. Without his assistance, our high quality contact tracing data would have to remain under-analyzed. As it was Dr. Rothenberg offered not only to provide computer data entry resources for our specially coded study sheets but, crucially, remained committed to helping analyze our data, which would have to be done in his spare time, a precious commodity in his life. (My favorite Rothenbergism: "I can only claim a constant state of overload".) His double duties, along with Woodhouse's departure for law school, help account for the sometimes long delay between field study termination in 1982 and completion of manuscripts. Balanced against departures, however, were arrivals, the most important being the appointment of Dr. John Muth as director of the health department in August 1980; he was to introduce and nurture a positive, supportive, and intelligent administration, a work environment context that lasted 16 years and took us through the difficult early years of the new sexually transmissible epidemic, AIDS.

A distinct advantage of our saturation contact tracing initiative was that it presented the opportunity to evaluate the differential importance of interviewing specific diagnostic categories. For example, it had long been orthodoxy that interviewing women whose infection was identified as a consequence of being a contact to a recently diagnosed man with symptomatic gonorrhea was futile, because her other contacts, if infected, were also likely to be symptomatic. Our data seriously undermined this assertion by demonstrating that nearly half of her other infected contacts were not only non-symptomatic, but likely to remain untreated in the community's gonorrhea reservoir.[21] This implied substantial accumulations of silently infected, untreated men in the local reservoir, since more than three-fifths of all women with gonorrhea fit this diagnostic category in Colorado Springs.

Importantly, availability of saturation contact tracing records presented the first ever opportunity to study gonorrhea transmission dynamics directly.[22] Previous efforts to derive estimates were based on indirect approaches: studies of male-to-female and female-to-male transmission rates, and analysis of disease trends and case reporting, to include accommodation of their usually considerable artifacts. Our direct empiric data quantified the contribution of different diagnostic categories of infected men: symptomatic, minimally symptomatic, and non-symptomatic, showing not only a steep gradient but, above all, the disproportionate impact on community gonorrhea transmission by non- and minimally-symptomatic cases. For example, we showed that nearly half of women with gonorrhea were infected by men without genital symptoms and that most (75%) of the other half were infected by symptomatic men *before* they had symptoms.[22] Hence the preponderance of women who acquired gonorrhea were infected by men with silent infection at the time of exposure.

An additional bonus of this direct evidence was to confirm that the CDC's indirectly derived estimate for the national gonorrhea burden was close to the mark—with actual estimated incidence outpacing reported cases by a factor of 1.7—but that its composition was the *reciprocal* of the CDC estimate: instead of the male-to-female ratio being 1.46:1, it was likelier to be 0.8:1 in the real world. This implied that national gonorrhea control initiatives in 1981 were failing to detect huge (nearly half a million) numbers of infected women.[22] Parenthetically, this analysis was my term paper for my advanced statistical analysis class at the University of Colorado, Colorado Springs in 1985 and, yes, I got an A.

Maybe the best contribution to gonorrhea transmission dynamics made possible by our saturation contact tracing data was the brainchild of Dr. Rothenberg's superlative analytic skills and dogged persistence to find definitive empiric evidence for Core Group Theory. His brilliant insight was to find contact tracing data *surrogates* for estimating the two critical parameters of gonorrhea transmission dynamics directly: the duration of gonorrhea's infectiousness in a community, and the extent of sexual mixing between different groups in that community. He invented the "force of infectivity", which refers to the amount of time that people with gonorrhea actually remain infectious and therefore potentially transmitting before their infections are medically intercepted.[23] And he introduced the terms "Self-Selection" and "Non Self-Selection"[23] to delineate the extent to which members of specific groups select their sexual contacts from within their own group, known in sociology as homophily. This exhaustive and meticulous analysis confirmed that gonorrhea is maintained by specific core groups within which intense transmission takes place and showed that community transmission is more related to interaction between subgroups than to the biology of infection.

Contact tracing's gift to VD surveillance

Assessment of the VD burden in society relies on periodic reports of numbers of diagnosed cases; these tallies are gathered by local health jurisdictions and customarily aggregated at the state and national levels. Artifacts and shortcomings in such reports make it difficult to interpret disease trends with confidence. For example, vagaries in case ascertainment and reporting in the private and quasi-private medical sectors, not to mention insufficient case descriptors—usually confined to sex, age, ethnicity, and location—make it challenging to discern transmission dynamics. Are cases currently being transmitted in gay or heterosexual populations? In both? If so, to what extent? Which subsets of these populations are now transmitting? Answers to these questions should guide focal application of control and prevention resources. This is where contact tracing data can provide reliable surveillance information. As we recently showed,[24] the key lies with small area (neighborhood level, where VD is actually being transmitted) analysis and then reporting each of these small area analyses to state and national health agencies, which could then distill patterns of transmission rather than simply count cases. Needless to say, these small area analyses depend on contact tracing data—the gift that keeps on giving.

Conclusion

A decade of assiduous gonorrhea contact tracing in Colorado Springs was largely responsible for revolutionizing the orthodox view of gonorrhea epidemiology and control. In summary, our empiric data provided direct evidence that gonorrhea was controllable in the absence of vaccines using case-finding measures. Federally sponsored demonstration projects to test contact tracing efficacy had been implemented several times between the early 1950s and the late 1970s.[3,10] Although details were never published, some reasons were advanced for failure of these endeavors to achieve incidence reduction; perhaps these projects were prematurely abandoned.[10] Our programmatic *idée fixe*—that men with silent infection were chiefly responsible for the maintenance of gonorrhea in communities—provided unassailable support for Pariser & Marino's contention that these men may be important in sustaining community transmission.[25] That these silently infected men were also important in the epidemiology of pre-pubertal gonorrhea was an unexpected bonus. And lastly, providing the initial and, eventually, the strongest and most detailed evidence to validate Core Group Theory was a notable achievement. A crucial contribution was our optimistic assessment that data-informed, rifled use of case-finding measures could substantially reduce gonorrhea incidence. After all, community gonorrhea control was our *raison d'être*.

In retrospect, though, our crowning achievement may well have been epidemiologic: providing the persuasive empiric evidence to buttress transmission dynamics theories, theories whose applicability go beyond the world of gonorrhea. And it is also here that we should recognize the long-term, dedicated contact tracers who made these exceptional data possible: Perry Bethea, Mark Brecher, Lynanne Phillips, Christopher Pratts, Donald Woodhouse, Helen P. Zimmerman, and me.

THREE

AIDS CONTROL & EPIDEMIOLOGY

"The essential thing was to save the greatest number of persons dying and being doomed to unending separation. And to do this, there was only one resource: to fight the plague. There was nothing admirable about this attitude: it was merely logical."

—Albert Camus: *The Plague* (1947)

Crisis on the horizon: The arrival of AIDS

The ending of the embedded gonorrhea-as-a-social-disease study[1] in June 1981 coincided with the beginning of a once-and-future social disease. For it was in that month that the CDC published reports of severe immunodeficiency in young, previously healthy homosexual men at UCLA's (my alma mater) hospital, a disease eventually called AIDS.[2]

Although I knew a lot about the exotic sexual, alcohol, and drug abuse lifestyles of adventurous gay men, my initial reaction on reading this new report was that this might be an outbreak caused by street drug contamination and that, therefore, it would soon go away. I neither suspected that the causative agent might be sexually transmissible nor sensed that AIDS-related work would consume most of my professional energies for the next three decades.

While epidemiologists and scientists at the CDC and in Europe were busy unraveling the causes of the AIDS outbreak, which they accomplished in the remarkably short time of a year and a half, we in Colorado Springs lived in a community that was distant from the bicoastal epicenters of what was quickly being recognized as an epidemic. Not only did the approaching epidemic, because it seemed to be moving inland slowly, give us time to complete the coding, data entry, and analysis of our recently completed gonorrhea contact tracing initiatives but, more importantly, afforded us lead time to think about how to handle it once it arrived.

Actually, we did not have to wait long before our first case surfaced in August 1982, a young African American woman newly arrived from Connecticut and hospitalized with painful cryptococcal meningitis. She was to be my first AIDS contact interview, requested by CDC in Atlanta, because there had been so few cases in women by then.

Her diagnosis was followed by a trickle of other cases, all in principally white gay or bisexual men, whom we interviewed for risk factor (but not sexual contacts) information for the CDC. We counseled persons with AIDS about transmission risk reduction; each was asked to (especially) refrain from donating blood, and to observe healthy habits to retard further damage to their immune system. As for their contacts, we gingerly recommended that they be told about possible contact with AIDS, so that exposed people might be more motivated to adopt safer sex and, if applicable, safer injection drug use behaviors. We thought this approach might work more effectively than letting at-risk persons be reached through impersonal AIDS prevention messages in the community. "Gingerly", because we knew that loose lips could sink ships, and because AIDS blood tests or treatments were not yet available. Our reasoning was that if contacts got upset and broke confidentiality through gossip ("loose lips"), AIDS patients would face discrimination and, worse, social isolation. In the beginning we chose not to do formal contact interviewing and tracing of named partners, not only because informed contacts would be placed in the anguishing position of not having a way to find out if they were infected, but also because we hoped that the frequent messages we disseminated on the ground in our gay communities would help fulfill our "duty to warn" responsibility. Simply put, until 1985, we almost exclusively relied on the message that if you were gay or bisexual you should behaviorally conduct yourself as if you were infected.

The pivotal year: 1985

For AIDS control, 1985 changed everything. Availability of the new AIDS virus (then called HTLV-III) antibody test in the Spring of 1985 and confirmation on the 25th of July that Rock Hudson had AIDS, transformed the public's perception of the disease from one afflicting marginal groups to the idea that "even nice people can get it". This was a momentous change and, probably, the most powerful catalyst to action since the beginning of the epidemic 4 years earlier. It was an open secret that the Reagan Administration's initial response to the epidemic had been callous;[3] among the cognoscenti, rumors circulated that the CDC's AIDS chief, Dr. Jim Curran, was frequently subjected to verbal abuse during his periodic visits to Washington to brief highly placed members of the Administration. Hudson not only, for the first time, gave AIDS an acceptable face but, more importantly, helped generate long-awaited substantial funding to fight this disease; a few days after his death on 2 October 1985, Congress allocated $221 million to find a cure.

By 1985, it had become clear to me that what was truly remarkable about AIDS was not how many, but how few, cases were occurring. Given how frequently people, especially gay men, were having sex, one should have expected far more cases if this virus were easy to transmit. As someone who was accustomed to seeing hundreds of STD cases every year, the reporting of only a dozen cases of AIDS in Colorado Springs between 1981 and 1985, led to my provisionally concluding that, however deadly this disease—and it was, because 11 of our 12 had died by the end of 1985—it was not likely to be easily transmitted. This impression was reinforced when, after the first six months of offering the HTLV-III antibody test, only 36 people, virtually all men providing histories of sex with other men, of injecting drug use, or both, had tested positive in Colorado Springs. These data, along with rough estimates of the number of gay/bisexual men and of injecting drug users in Colorado Springs, allowed me to venture a crude projection[4] that about 1665 people would be cumulatively identified as being positive by the year 2000. (The actual number[5] at the end of 1999 was 1318.) The other, and more crucial, observation that helped generate this modest and surprisingly accurate projection was AIDS' stubbornly conservative epidemiologic boundaries: reports from all over the United States consistently indicated that AIDS was not breaking out of the major groups initially described: men who have sex with men, injecting drug users, hemophiliacs and, to a lesser extent, Haitians, unkindly referred to as the "4-H Club" (homosexuals, heroin addicts, hemophiliacs, and Haitians). In my view, based on admittedly limited experience, the few infected heterosexual women reporting no classic risk factor were very likely those who practiced receptive anal intercourse. The fact that there had been many opportunities for people in other groups, principally non-drug injecting heterosexuals, to be sexually exposed to infected bisexual or street drug injecting men and women (especially prostitutes and especially in New York City) during the first few years of the epidemic, and that by 1985 there were so few cases among these people argued that, absent the high risk behaviors of unprotected receptive anal sex or use of contaminated injecting equipment, the chances of getting AIDS were remote. (Again unkindly AIDS was, at the time, referred to by mostly unsympathetic lay people as an acronym for "Anally Inserted Death Sentence".)

Desperately seeking AIDS cases in heterosexuals

From the CDC's point of view, these were ugly facts. Jim Curran's allegedly negative experiences with the powers that be in Washington suggests that political sympathy and continued funding to fight this behaviorally confined epidemic might well hinge on the perception that AIDS was crossing over into heterosexual populations. And then came the cavalry to the rescue—coincidentally at almost the same time Rock Hudson died. Researchers at Walter Reed Army Medical Center in Washington DC reported, in the prestigious *Journal of the American Medical Association (JAMA)*, that about 30 percent of their AIDS-virus infected soldiers did not have the recognized risk factors, concluding that they had probably acquired infection heterosexually, most likely via contact with prostitutes.[6] In their surveillance scheme the CDC had classified such cases into a temporary category called NIR (No Identified Risk); the 30% rate reported by Walter Reed researchers was a stunning 5 times greater than the national average. How to explain it? This is where we came in, much to the chagrin of the Armed Forces and, possibly, the CDC.

Years of experience interviewing soldiers with syphilis diagnosed at Fort Carson's Preventive Medicine Section had taught us that soldiers admitting a history of homosexual sex or of injecting drug use was not uncommon, and that such pejorative behaviors were likelier to be revealed to civilian workers than to their Army employers. Again by coincidence, the timing could not have been more perfect because, a few days after publication of the Walter Reed findings, Colorado became the first State to require mandatory reporting of HTLV-III (by now called HIV) infection on 1 November 1985. This gave us the opportunity to test our a priori conviction that risk factors for soldiers were no different from those of civilians. Our data eventually proved us right; we were able to interview 20 of the 22 HIV/AIDS cases reported by Fort Carson during the ensuing 12 months, and to detail the striking differences in risk factors being revealed to us compared to those revealed to Army medical personnel. Not only was our risk factor information the inverse of that obtained by Army interviewers, but it almost exactly mirrored the national experience.

Our results appeared in *JAMA*[7] in Spring 1987 and created a furor, especially at the Pentagon and at Fort Carson. Part of the anger was directed at the article's title, "Lying to military physicians about risk factors for HIV infections", which the military must have viewed as a cheeky affront to members of their community. Nor did they know that it was the *JAMA* editors who changed our dry, neutral title to a more in-your-face one. That at least seven of the nine blood donors among the 20 soldiers we interviewed revealed risk factors that should have prompted self-exclusion from the donor pool was also an embarrassment for the Army. As a consequence of our publishing these results without first letting them know—clearly my fault— authorities at Fort Carson not only denied us continued access to their HIV patients, but also delayed reporting HIV cases. This was a clever (and successful) Fabian tactic, because by the time these Army cases were reported, these HIV-infected soldiers would have been re- assigned elsewhere, well beyond our interviewing reach.

My doubting claims of HIV "heterosexual transmission" in the absence of rigorous evidence started as a cottage industry in about 1983; as we shall see later, it has continued unabated since. My objection to jumping to conclusions without valid evidence sprung from my extensive experience interviewing patients with syphilis, especially closeted gay men in west Los Angeles neighborhoods. Many had lied, hiding behind stereotypic claims of sexual exposure to anonymous prostitutes in Tijuana, Mexico. Interviewer skill and, above all, persistence in challenging the patient's prefabricated story were the best predictors of interviewing success. My first *published* objection to jumping to conclusions without valid evidence suggested a way to indirectly gauge the veracity of such patients' stories: do additional blood tests, based on the idea that "Patients may lie, but blood doesn't". My suggestion was published in *JAMA* 8 months prior to the above article about risk factors in Fort Carson servicemen.[8] It consisted of recommending testing HIV/AIDS patients who deny recognized risk factors for several predictive markers of risk: antibody to cytomegalovirus, to Hepatitis-B virus, and to the syphilis spirochete. Such markers were, respectively, 2 times, 9 times, and 14 times more common in homosexuals than in heterosexuals. Not only would such actuarial information improve case classification validity but, more importantly, could discourage announcements of unsubstantiated, speculative patterns of HIV transmission in the United States. Such announcements might needlessly worry segments of the population at minimal risk and, crucially, cause distortions in the allocation of scarce control resources.

To backtrack a little, before our 2 publications appeared in *JAMA*, the CDC had decided, in the summer of 1986, to reclassify certain AIDS cases as heterosexually acquired, specifically those diagnosed in patients from Third World countries. This reclassification, from "No Risk Identified" to "Heterosexual Transmission", was done ex cathedra, in the absence of valid evidence. For all anyone knew, infection might have been acquired via contaminated sharps in health care settings; inadequate sterilization of medical equipment was a common occurrence in the reclassified cases' countries of origin. So why jump to conclusions by inference only, without quality evidence? This scientifically-questionable and, most likely, politically-motivated decision helped fuel the perception that AIDS was moving into heterosexual populations. The media lost little time capitalizing on this perceived threat; soon alarmist media reports became rampant, certainly spreading faster than AIDS. Media concern had been conspicuously absent during the years that marginalized populations were reported to be at risk.[9] It turns out that, to the media at least, some people counted for more than others.

This alarmist media campaign started in 1986 and lasted many years. And it played right into the hands not only of the public health establishment, which had been fighting so long and so hard for adequate funding with only modest results, but into the hands of many other groups. In a refreshingly non-alarmist editorial published on 3 February 1987, the *New York Times* summarized the likely interests of other stakeholders: "…the chief interpreters of the data want them to reflect their own messages. Public health experts see a unique chance to reduce all sexually transmitted diseases. Medical researchers demand $1 billion in new Federal spending against AIDS, hoping to refurbish their laboratories. Government epidemiologists, seeking to protect homosexuals and drug addicts, fear the Reagan Administration may acquire the notion that these are the only people at risk. Moralists see a heaven-sent chance to preach fire, brimstone and restricted sex. Homosexuals have no desire to carry the stigma of AIDS alone. With so many experts dramatizing the epidemic, it's little wonder that those who depend on their advice are coming to believe that AIDS is already as rampant as influenza."

Voila! From then on, cascades of money would be allocated to fight HIV in the developed world and, subsequently, in Third World countries, especially in sub-Saharan Africa. I genuinely doubt that generous allocations for HIV research and for HIV control would have been made available absent the perceived imminent threat to heterosexuals here or elsewhere in the world.

Contemporaneously, *The Atlantic* published a lengthy article in its February 1987 issue by Katie Leishman, who was trying to convey a sense for the future of the AIDS epidemic in heterosexuals. Its title suggested her inclination: "Heterosexuals and AIDS: The second stage of the epidemic". This article led to my first published attempt to counter budding alarmist media reports with epidemiologic evidence indicating that rapid transmission in U.S. heterosexuals was unlikely to occur. I concluded my counter article by saying that rather than facing an imminent flood, heterosexuals were probably facing a drippy faucet, using this metaphor to convey the idea that heterosexual transmission in American communities was unlikely to be self-sustaining.[10] By exaggerating the magnitude of the AIDS threat to the general population, the media was instilling fears out of proportion to what was indicated by the available scientific evidence. Above all, I expressed my concern about the media's generally uncritical analysis of AIDS reports, and about the virtual absence of dissent in media reports concerning the AIDS threat to the general population. Absence of dissent in mainstream media was a reality that extended, ironically, to my manuscript, for it was rejected by both *The Atlantic* and *Harper's Magazine*. It was eventually published in a fringe journal: *Critique: A Journal of Conspiracies & Metaphysics*.[10] As uncomfortable as any association with conspiracy frames of mind made me, I consented to its appearing there, not because I expected broad readership, but because I wanted to be able to say, many years later: "Told you so". Indeed, more than a quarter-century after publication of my dissenting manuscript, a heterosexual epidemic—meaning one sustained by penile-vaginal sex—has yet to materialize in the developed world. Mine was not the only dissenting voice. There were a few other observers who published pieces, mainly letters to the editor or brief commentaries in medical or public health journals, doubting that the second stage of the epidemic would occur in heterosexual populations. Their comments failed to persuade readers, especially those in a position to influence policy. It seemed clear to me by the late 1980s that fear- rather than science-based assessments would continue to win the hearts and minds of both professional and lay people. (I comment at length on the "heterosexual" AIDS epidemics of sub-Saharan Africa in Chapter 7.)

The fact that I failed to find evidence of AIDS spreading rapidly in heterosexual *populations* did not mean that I did not believe HIV infection could be transmitted "heterosexually" in certain *individuals*. Early in the AIDS epidemic I suggested that facilitating factors, specifically the loss of epithelial tissue integrity caused by syphilis ulcers[11] in—or by infections or trauma to—the genitals, could facilitate transmission during what was a very inefficient way to transmit HIV: penile-vaginal sex. Although the idea that transmission could be facilitated by loss of epithelial integrity had been suggested the year before,[12] my contribution was to offer plausible empiric evidence.[11] In addition, because syphilis and other genital infections were more common in black Americans than in other U.S. populations, I urged that special public health attention be devoted to prevention efforts in black communities to head off AIDS epidemics in their midst.[11] (Recall that this was at a time when AIDS was viewed principally as a problem of white gay men.) No such prevention priority was formally advocated by the CDC until 20 years later.[13–14]

CDC studies of AIDS heterosexual transmission:
Colorado Springs' participation

Over time, the CDC became increasingly interested in delineating the sexual (in addition to the intravenous drug use) epidemiology of AIDS virus infection in heterosexual populations. A study by Peterman and his CDC colleagues, initiated in mid-1984 and conducted in 1985–1986, attempted to elucidate virus transmissibility in heterosexuals by studying couples consisting of a transfusion-associated infected person and of the other reporting no known risk. This study confirmed intra-couple sexual transmission, but revealed sharply varying transmission probabilities, an enigma which remains unsolved [15] (Personal communication with Peterman 28 July 2014).

To develop a clearer sense of transmission dynamics on the population, and not simply intra-couple, level CDC proposed assessing AIDS virus prevalence in people inferred to be high-risk heterosexuals, such as female prostitutes and intravenous drug users (later labeled "injecting drug users"). On the same day in July 1985 that Rock Hudson, a gay man, finally admitted his AIDS diagnosis of the previous year, the Federal Register announced availability of funding for cooperative agreements with the CDC to study AIDS virus prevalence and associated risk factors in U.S. prostitutes. This was to be Phase I (CDC Project 72). Five high-priority applications were funded. Two more agencies, the health departments in Las Vegas and in Colorado Springs, agreed to join the study without Federal funding. I volunteered, because I knew we would succeed in enrolling prostitutes locally, not only because we had earned their trust since the late 1960s, but also because we had been pleasantly surprised by their cooperation when asked to take the recently (mid-1985) available AIDS virus antibody test. (The stereotypic response was: "Of course we should be tested!") Starting in May 1986, we recruited 71 (5% of the nearly 1400 recruited nationally) prostitutes during the one-year enrollment period; one was HIV-antibody positive. National prevalence in recruited prostitutes was principally associated with intravenous drug use and tended to mirror local HIV prevalence in other women.[16] Although data about anal intercourse had been collected and were subsequently reported for an analysis of these prostitutes' Hepatitis-B risks,[17] its probable association with AIDS virus infection was not reported. I suspect that this "oversight" was deliberate and due to political reasons within the CDC. In any event, this would not be the last instance of CDC's reluctance to associate HIV infection with anal intercourse in heterosexuals.[16,18]

Phase II of this CDC-initiated study of prostitutes was funded and awarded to us (CDC Project 90); it was designed to study the socio-sexual networks of female prostitutes and of intravenous drug users locally, in an attempt to see how high-risk heterosexuals were linked to others in the community via social, sexual, and drug using behaviors. This pioneering study, conducted between 1987 and 1991, was the first prospective study of the influence of network structure on the propagation of an infectious disease and is presented in Chapter 6. For our immediate purposes, I note that no HIV infection in either female prostitutes or intravenous drug users or in their contacts was linked to penile-vaginal exposures during more than a decade of prospective observation.[19]

> "He who desires and acts not, breeds pestilence"
>
> —William Blake

Contact tracing for HIV/AIDS in Colorado Springs: 1985–2000

Our interviewing HIV-infected soldiers at Fort Carson starting in November of 1985 was part of our newly implemented approach to HIV/AIDS epidemiology and control. Now that we had reliable AIDS virus antibody tests, plus a state health regulation mandating reports of HIV infection (AIDS proper had been reportable since 1983) and funding to set up an Alternate Test Site (ATS), I decided that it would be useful to do contact interviews on all newly diagnosed HIV/AIDS patients in Colorado Springs. The ATS was devised by national public health authorities to discourage high-risk people, especially gay men and intravenous drug users, from donating blood to find out their HIV antibody status. The person who accepted the challenge to run the ATS and to implement HIV contact tracing was the experienced nurse who had done the intensive interviews on selected women with gonorrhea between 1976 and 1978,[20] Lynanne Phillips. She had resigned her position in June 1978 when her daughter was born, and had subsequently worked with a private health organization for the preceding five years. Like the rest of our STD program staff, she was comfortable dealing with all people in high-risk STD/HIV populations.

In 1985, we were among the very few public health programs in the world to perform contact tracing for HIV infection; public health workers in Minnesota, Sweden, and Sheffield (England) probably started at about the same time we did in Colorado Springs. My reasoning at the time was that contact tracing was a time-honored tool to control communicable diseases and that contact tracing for HIV should be used, at least until empiric evidence indicated it was not effective.[21] I was willing to try anything that would retard HIV transmission in Colorado Springs, as long as it was ethical and acceptable to patients. I knew in advance that it would be acceptable not only because the first few interviews done had proved uneventful, but because contact interviewing and contact tracing were inherently voluntary activities: if the patient did not want to cooperate, there was nothing we could do. For the first several years, contact tracing was clearly not an endeavor advocated by the larger AIDS public health community. Their view was that it would be an ineffective intervention and an unnecessary civil intrusion ("bedroom police").[22] They believed that because HIV was a lethal infection affecting principally stigmatized people who practiced negatively viewed sexual behaviors such as anal intercourse, contact tracing would have too much potential for discrimination. As well, this perception occurred in context of fears that the government would be keeping lists of members of these stigmatized groups to the detriment of their right to privacy. Another important concern was that, in the absence of effective treatments or vaccines, contact tracing would not be efficacious. Contact tracing was generally opposed by AIDS activists, by civil libertarians, and (disappointingly) by many public health workers, who were often influenced by political correctness and by not wanting to offend strident constituencies.[22]

Our view was that even if contact tracing only consisted of focal counseling to discourage further transmission and to retard disease progression, this intervention would be of greater benefit to them and to society at large than doing nothing. By 1988, the view that contact tracing could be useful was formally endorsed by CDC, which now encouraged public health workers to evaluate its efficacy.[23] We chose the right course initially not because we were smart or wise but because, unlike more highly placed public health authorities who were often divorced from realities on the ground, we were in daily contact with our high-risk populations. We knew them, and their attitudes vis-a-vis public health interventions, well.

During the first 15 years of contact tracing for HIV/AIDS in Colorado Springs we interviewed nearly 700 cases; they helped identify, directly and indirectly, about 1900 contacts. Interventions with these people may have contributed to the 90% decline in reported HIV cases in Colorado Springs between 1986 and the end of the century, from 43 to 5 cases per 100,000, probably by selectively fragmenting high transmission networks (breaking up highly connected network regions).[24] Admittedly, steep incidence decline was most likely due to substantial reductions in risky behaviors by gay men rather than to contact tracing's ability to fragment networks, although the latter undoubtedly occurred. Of importance as well was the non-adversarial relationship between members of the highest-risk populations and our health department, a trust that had been nurtured in context of mutual respect since the late 1960s. Presumably, this trust and our constant presence in their lives—in local media, in our clinics, in contact tracing space, and in gay venues,[25] served as relentless reminders to pay attention to safer behaviors.

Yet, the most important epidemiologic result from this sustained HIV contact tracing endeavor was completely unexpected. And a wonderful surprise it was. In 2000, after having analyzed the network connections of nearly 4,600 chlamydia cases and their 7,400 contacts reported in Colorado Springs between 1996 and 1999, we were able to directly demonstrate, for the first time anywhere, the relationship between sexual network structure and STD epidemic phase (See Chapter 4). Encouraged by this result, we decided to similarly analyze the network structure of the nearly 700 HIV/AIDS cases and 1,900 linked contacts who had been reported between 1985 and 1999. Again, a direct connection between network structure and epidemic phase (whether an infectious disease is waxing or waning, as we shall see later) was empirically demonstrated.[24]

More importantly, by focusing on the earliest and largest connected component (a network region where everyone can be shown to be connected, directly or indirectly to everyone else; this one consisted of

250 unique individuals), our brilliant resident network analyst Steve Muth was able, using a stepwise reduction technique, to remove the wheat from the chaff, as it were, and expose our community's core HIV transmitters (here represented as the persons connected by thicker lines).

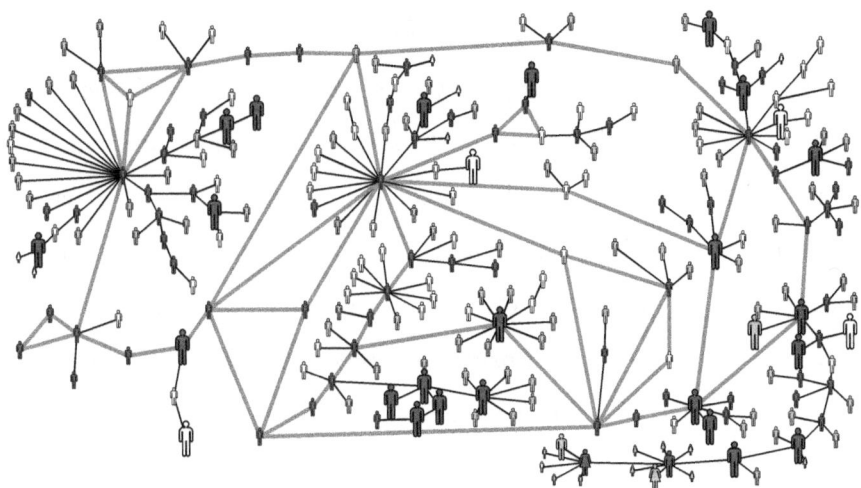

LEGEND (MSM=men who have sex with men; IDU=person using IV drugs)

N=250	MSM & IDU	IDU		MSM	Other	
	M (28)	M (2)	F (2)	M (202)	M (4)	F (12)
HIV negative (63)	(4)	(0)	(0)	(53)	(1)	(5)
HIV positive (96)	(23)	(1)	(1)	(71)	(0)	(0)
HIV unknown (91)	(1)	(1)	(1)	(78)	(3)	(7)

Figure 1. Network of sexual and injecting drug-use connections of persons in the early phase of HIV transmission in Colorado Springs

Original illustration by Steve Muth, October 2015, and is based on our article in *Sexually Transmitted Infections*.[24]

This network analysis technique removes linear branching patterns, leaving only the cyclically connected ones—meaning terminal branches were pared, revealing only the densely-interconnected nodes; these 39 cyclically-connected people (nodes), four-fifths of whom were HIV-positive gay men, including five who were also injecting drug users, are viewed as the inner core of transmitting individuals forming "ground zero" for HIV propagation locally.[24] In brief, our local HIV epidemic was most likely initially ignited in the social spaces of gay injecting drug users. "Completely unexpected" because none of us foresaw that our HIV contact tracing data could act as an epidemiologic Hubble Telescope, taking us as close to the initial Big Bang of HIV transmission in Colorado Springs as could ever be done. This is yet another instance of contact tracing's power to provide epidemiologic results greater than the sum of its parts.

HIV contact tracing: the national mood

Regrettably, CDC's 1988 recommendation to implement contact tracing,[23] which was now called partner notification (PN), largely fell on reluctant ears. By this time, the HIV public health climate had undergone momentous changes, mostly under the relentless pressure from AIDS activists, who were highly politicized gay men. Such activists early argued forcefully, nay vociferously, for public health-exempt status in HIV control efforts, objecting specifically to implementation of standard public health interventions such as mandatory name reporting, contact tracing, closing of high-transmission venues, and behavior restrictions. As I wrote elsewhere: "In their stead came civil liberties-inspired, client-centered, community organization-mediated initiatives encouraging anonymity. Oversight of HIV/AIDS control initiatives shifted, starting in the late 1980s, from public health workers to behavioral scientists, then clinicians, and then politically motivated activists. Accompanying this transfer of actual public health power was a subtle shift, pregnant with fate, in the underlying philosophy, from community orientation to focus on customer service—in brief, public health by plebiscite. This, in my opinion, is the principal reason for the pro forma support accorded to PN by those who control the local community response to HIV/AIDS, despite its endorsement by the public health establishment. Those in positions of authority are professionally disinclined to implement it because, likelier than not, they subscribe to the "patient-autonomy model".[26]

To a disappointing extent, the history of the AIDS epidemic has been the history of clashing professional paradigms. As Richards and Rathburn observe, "the patient autonomy model that underlies personal health care is incompatible with the subrogation of individual interests that is necessary for effective public health, which puts the community's interests before those of the individual patient...[and] rejects the patient's right to have sole control of his/her treatment."[27]

Opposition to contact tracing started in the early 1980s, with opponents arguing that in the absence of a test, there was no compelling reason to do it. Once the test became available in 1985, opposition shifted to fears that contact tracing would lead to government agencies' compilation of lists of homosexuals. The next objection was that, in the absence of effective treatment, notifying partners would needlessly anguish them and perhaps lead to an increase in suicides.[26] With the arrival in 1987 of AZT, the first effective and widely distributed treatment for AIDS, the next ground for objection was that contact tracing would be inordinately expensive,[28] an argument we seriously undermined with empiric information.[21] For the record, none of these objections was supported by experience or by data, only by misperception and ideology. For us, a crucial datum was that, in Colorado, only one-fifth of the partners of HIV positive cases were notified by the infected person.[29] Who, then, would notify the other four-fifths of partners? The unfortunate consequence of these public health climate changes was that, as late as the year 2001, only about one-third of newly identified HIV cases in the United States were being interviewed for contact tracing purposes.[30] How does one measure what we've lost because of this misguided reluctance?

Marginalized and homeless populations

To develop a sense for the prevalence of high-risk behaviors and for unmet HIV prevention needs in marginalized populations in Colorado Springs, we conducted field outreach to enroll homeless persons, out-of-treatment drug addicts, and mentally ill street persons.[31] In brief, we found that such persons had been exposed to offers of prevention services and had previously been HIV tested (69%), were local residents (74%) but frequently homeless, were willing to participate in our study (95%), and commonly reported high-risk behaviors such as injecting drug use (24%), receptive anal intercourse (33% of women; 8% of men), or having multiple sex partners in the previous six months (25%). The low HIV prevalence noted (1% of participants) was associated with social isolation: most were un(der)employed (96%), homeless (44%), unattached (85%), and used drugs alone (44%). In brief, such social attributes made for fragmented HIV risk networks where opportunities for sustained HIV transmission would be dampened. This study thus provided additional empiric evidence for the importance of network structure in the propagation—or lack of it—of HIV in communities, despite the substantial presence of risk behaviors. Network structure may well be destiny.

Use of legal means in Colorado to discourage preventable HIV transmission

Nationally, reluctance to apply previously acceptable public health tools extended to application of legal measures to protect communities from preventable HIV transmission. With communicable diseases, public health's first responsibility is to protect the uninfected. In 1987, a small part of new public health legislation in Colorado aimed to revise existing statutes dealing with isolation and quarantine. Specifically, procedures were promulgated to deal with HIV-infected people who were endangering others through irresponsible behavior. Once efforts to obtain voluntary compliance had failed, the following procedures were to be applied step-wise starting from the least restrictive one. Failure to comply with any level was grounds for invoking the next and more restrictive step: 1) Intensive counseling about dangerous behaviors; 2) issuance of a Cease & Desist Order, with the health officer prohibiting specific behaviors; 3) Issuance of a Restriction Order, where the health officer restricts a person's opportunity to expose others (e.g., prohibiting an infected prostitute from appearing in prostitution areas); and 4) Issuance of an Order of Compliance, where the health officer turns over enforcement of specific proscriptions to a court.[32] Our program took these measures seriously and invoked them without hesitation whenever reliable information about misbehaviors on the part of an HIV-infected person was strongly suspected or known to be endangering other people's health. We were also fortunate to have our health department director, Dr. John Muth, and the director of the Colorado Department of Health, Dr. Tom Vernon, unequivocally support implementation of these procedures as they arose, given adequate evidence of the accused's misbehaviors. Details about management of the first twenty HIV-infected people on whom these procedures were serially applied, including an illustrative subset of four detailed case reports, were published in 1993,[32] to my knowledge the only such report in the literature.

The tragedy of the AIDS epidemic in the early years:

premature death

The gonorrhea-as-a-social-disease study,[1] which spanned the first half of 1981, also presented us with the opportunity to develop a sense for mortality in a population at high risk for AIDS: homosexual men diagnosed with gonorrhea in Colorado Springs during those 6 months. These 69 young men (average age 24 years) were sexually active in the pre-AIDS awareness era. We assessed mortality status exactly 20 years later using the Social Security Death Index, comparing them to a one-third random sample consisting of 131 heterosexual men diagnosed with gonorrhea (average age 23.4 years) during the same interval in Colorado Springs. Twenty-one (30.4%) homosexual and 7 (5.3%) heterosexual men were ascertained as having died between 1981 and 2000. The former died at an average age of 37.9 years, a datum virtually identical to that of the 315 homosexual men in the Colorado Springs database known to have died of AIDS (37.7 years) during those 20 years. The heterosexual comparison men died at an average age of 40.9 years. We confirmed that, of the 21 homosexuals who died and for whom cause of death was available, ninety percent had died of AIDS.[33] The observation that 30% of homosexual men with gonorrhea in Colorado Springs during the first half of 1981—an area eventually assessed as having a low AIDS burden—are known to have died during the ensuing 20 years is notable. Whether these homosexual men acquired HIV elsewhere before moving to or from Colorado Springs is not knowable; yet this fact takes little from the stark realization that such men were 6 times more likely to die young than their heterosexual counterparts.

Discerning the magnitude and direction of the HIV epidemic using hard data

Our observing so few cases during the 1980s was not the only major clue to our view that the HIV epidemic would neither rapidly expand nor seriously threaten the general heterosexual population. In its sexual transmission form, HIV resembled syphilis, not only because it infected essentially the same populations (gay men, prostitutes, brown minority heterosexuals), but also because it was neither highly infectious nor spread very rapidly. Hence there were always far fewer cases of syphilis than, say, gonorrhea being transmitted every year. In its blood-borne transmission form, HIV resembled Hepatitis-B in its transmission modes and in that it was also highly confined in risk groups similar to those affecting HIV-infected people. Our sense was that, after some time, enough transmission of HIV infection in these circumscribed groups would lead to the "preemption effect": transmission opportunities eventually wane because the number of available susceptible people (those not already infected) decline over time. By the late 1980s what I inferred from this perspective was that the HIV epidemic would soon implode. At the time, such a projection ran completely counter to virtually all assessments and public messages about the future of the AIDS epidemic.[34-35]

Because I knew that there would not be particularly brisk demand for this view in either the public health literature or in the media, I decided to seek publication in the local county government newsletter. Once again, my intention was to be able to tell folks years hence: "Told you so". This short article, called "The Coming AIDS Implosion" appeared in the March/April 1991 issue.[36] It projected that there would be far fewer HIV-infected people in the nation by the year 2000 than there were in 1985 (estimated at about 700,000). My projection was based on 3 observations: that HIV was difficult to acquire; that the high-risk populations were presently implementing substantial behavior changes, suggesting that fewer and fewer people would be getting infected during the decade; and that HIV infection had high mortality. I estimated that about 1,300,000 people in the United States would have ever been infected by the year 2000 and that, because I also estimated that 900,000 of them would have died by then, only about 400,000 HIV-infected people would still be living. Mine was evidently an underestimate, because the "true" number of people living with HIV by the year 2000 was officially estimated by the CDC at between 800,000 and 1,200,000, 2 to 3 times greater than my estimate. Part of the reason for my underestimate was innate optimism; I've always had trouble evaluating situations pessimistically. A probably more influential part of the reason was availability, starting in 1996, of powerful medications capable of significantly prolonging life. (For example, death rates plummeted by 83% during the latter part of the 1990s in Colorado Springs.[37]) HIV infection was no longer a short-term death sentence. Although the contention that the HIV epidemic in the

79

United States would implode did not materialize, whatever the reasons, the contention that it would not spread rapidly as often predicted turned out to be correct. The HIV epidemic not only slowed considerably during the 1990s, but actually stabilized at much lower levels than the usual dire predictions implied. Nevertheless, implosion was not the correct prediction for the nation, with all of its implications for vainglorious bragging rights!

Yet did "implosion" apply to the observed epidemic trajectory locally? Probably. The data collected in Colorado Springs from the beginning of the epidemic through 1992 support this view; they were published the following year under the suggestive title of "AIDS in Colorado Springs: is there an epidemic?"[38] These data were comprehensively collected, via intense surveillance of HIV/AIDS infection in blood/plasma donation centers and in private, quasi-private, public, and military clinics; via intensive testing in high-risk populations (homosexuals, prostitutes, injecting drug users—often including their partners); and via routine HIV contact tracing. Nearly 850,000 HIV antibody tests were done between 1985 and 1992, in a community with a 1990 Census total population of 400,000. These strong data clearly indicated that HIV infection was neither widespread nor spreading more widely (read: into the general population) nor rapidly increasing. Indeed close examination over time of average ages at 1) initial HIV infection; 2) first report; 3) AIDS diagnosis; and 4) AIDS death suggested that incidence was at least stable and most likely decreasing and that death would soon exceed cases of new HIV transmission.[38]

Specifically, the age distribution of reported cases was slowly increasing, suggesting ageing of an historically infected population, rather than fresh transmission in young populations, and also undermining the au courant assertion that teenagers were the next high-risk group. Crucially, the ratio of newly reported cases to death was dramatically decreasing, from 14.2:1 (128 HIV positives to 9 deaths) during 1986 to 2.7:1 (95 HIV positives to 35 deaths) in 1992. This trend continued through the mid-1990s, when effective treatments became available;[37] after 1996, greater survival of HIV-infected people would serve to stop the implosion and reverse the decreasing trend recorded during the 10 years between 1986 and 1995 in Colorado Springs.

Conscientious application of time-honored public health measures in Colorado Springs to diagnose and treat the HIV epidemic not only provided an accurate picture of its magnitude and direction, but also had palpable impact. Although the former claim is easier to associate with solid empiric evidence than the latter, it is reasonable to suppose that our interventions—sustained, focal education efforts in high-risk groups; continuous outreach in high-risk settings;[25,31, 39–40] assiduous HIV contact tracing; condom distribution (NOT at taxpayer expense), and individual counseling in both civilian and military VD clinics, as well as in HIV testing sites—contributed substantially to the behavior changes that must underlie the spectacular decrease in reported HIV cases during the last 15 years of the 20th century. I estimate that nearly 2,000,000 condoms were distributed by our programs in Colorado

Springs between 1987 and 1999, at a cost of about $120,000.[41] And this is not to mention the substantial number of HIV prevention presentations made by members of our STD/HIV programs to lower risk groups and the general population: nearly 1,200 presentations, averaging about 40 listeners, for an estimated overall attendance of 50,000 persons during that same time interval.[41] This process presumably also occurred in other American communities. What is especially gratifying to note is that meticulous documentation of empiric data to support our diagnosis and treatment of the HIV epidemic in Colorado Springs represents a possibly unique achievement. I am not aware of any published reports providing the breadth and depth of detail we obtained to elucidate the trajectory of the HIV epidemic in a single community over a long period. It is also a fine testament to the power and relevance of traditional public health measures to control communicable disease.

FOUR

CHLAMYDIA CONTROL & EPIDEMIOLOGY

The emergence of chlamydia control: In the shadow of AIDS

Although chlamydia, a genital disease similar to gonorrhea, was first shown to be sexually transmitted in the early years of the 20th century, it wasn't until the late 1960s that reliable—but expensive—culture tests were developed. They were used experimentally during the first half of the 1970s to show that chlamydia was a common infection, probably more common than the then #1 reportable disease in the United States, gonorrhea. At the time, though, few people had heard of it or knew much about its epidemiology. As I wrote more than twenty years ago: "Chlamydia needs a press agent. Although we are about 100 times more likely to get infected with it than HIV, chlamydia has not yet received the recognition it deserves. Most people have never heard of it. It escapes public recognition much the same way it is able to escape some of our immune defenses: by hiding. On the individual level, it hides inside the cells of the genital tract; on the community level, it hides in the shadow of AIDS."[1]

Chlamydia control efforts in communities awaited not only better press but, above all, availability of affordable and less cumbersome tests than the gold standard McCoy cell culture. Though modestly reliable and relatively inexpensive tests arrived in the early 1980s, our program was not able to afford them until the late 1980s. Although the primary reason for implementing a chlamydia control program was to prevent infertility in stereotypic chlamydia patients (very young women), an additional consideration was the received wisdom that genital infections rendered people more susceptible to HIV infection if sexually exposed. Hence, during the second half of 1987, we initiated a pilot chlamydia screening program in our health department's prenatal, family planning, and VD, clinics. Except for prenatal clinic, in which all patients were screened, only selected high-risk patients in the other 2 clinics were screened, which resulted in about half of patients being tested. Chlamydia-positive patients were occasionally formally interviewed for contacts; initially, they were most often counseled to refer their own partners to medical examination.

Contact tracing for chlamydia: Enter Helen L. Zimmerman-Rogers

Beginning in January 1988, having successfully obtained funding in late 1987 for additional full-time help, we implemented chlamydia contact tracing for cases diagnosed in all health department medical clinics. The newly funded contact tracer specifically placed in charge of chlamydia control was Helen P. Zimmerman's daughter, Helen L. Zimmerman-Rogers. At about the same time, we encouraged the military's VD clinics to screen for chlamydia infection and to formally interview positives to identify their sexual partners; happily, staff at these clinics complied. Cases diagnosed in the quasi-private (e.g., Planned Parenthood and community health clinics) and private medical settings were not sought out for interview, because chlamydia was not yet a reportable disease in Colorado; indeed in the mid-1980s, only about half of American states required notification of chlamydia cases to public health officers.[2]

It did not take long after implementation of chlamydia screening in our VD clinic to notice that patients with chlamydia were different from those with gonorrhea; the former were seemingly younger and more often white than the latter, who tended to be a bit older and more often black. I decided that, as long as we had adequate field contact tracing help, we should take this opportunity to use it, as we had in the past with gonorrhea, to develop a clearer sense of community chlamydia prevalence, patient characteristics, and transmission patterns than we currently had. We also needed to know to what extent our impressionistic observations might be artifactual. In addition, having recently taken a year course in statistical analysis at the local branch of the University of Colorado provided an opportunity to enter our data, sanitized of personal identifiers, into the university's powerful VAX 8600 (Digital Equipment Co.) computer, and to use their SPSS-X statistical package. Ease of analysis, coupled with assistance from my statistics professor, Dr. Richard Dukes, were important inducements for implementing a formal epidemiologic study.

Epidemiologic differences between chlamydia and gonorrhea

What truly puzzled me was why two sexually transmitted infections that appeared to be twins would seemingly affect different people in the community. After all, both were transmitted the same way and preferentially infected the same tissue—columnar epithelium—in the same anatomical sites: the genitals, the anus, and the conjunctiva (inside of eyelids). The main difference was that gonorrhea colonized the *inter*cellular, and chlamydia the *intra*cellular, spaces. Once again, it was our program which provided the empiric evidence to confirm that these 2 clinically similar STD indeed had a remarkably dissimilar community form.[3]

Contact interviews of both gonorrhea and chlamydia cases diagnosed in our health department clinics during 1988, coupled with field follow-up of named sexual contacts indicated that, in Colorado Springs, chlamydia cases were on average 2 years younger than gonorrhea cases; that the majority of chlamydia cases were diagnosed in whites (in men 62% v. 40% for gonorrhea cases; in women 60% v. 47% for gonorrhea). Geographic case distribution was diffuse for chlamydia, and highly concentrated for gonorrhea; there was only 40% geographic overlap between the 2 STD. Diagnostic overlap was also strikingly dissimilar: only 9 percent of chlamydia patients also had gonorrhea at diagnosis, compared to the 31 percent of gonorrhea patients with dual infection. It was as if these fraternal twin microbes travelled in different universes. In addition, each disease was differently expressed clinically, with chlamydia being much less likely to proclaim its presence via symptoms than gonorrhea. For example, while 85 percent of men with gonorrhea had urethral symptoms, only 54 percent of men with chlamydia did. We consequently speculated that silent chlamydial infection might be largely responsible for its differential socio-geographic distribution in the community.[3] Moreover, the epidemiologic picture for sexual partners mirrored that of cases. This should not have been surprising, because people usually mix with their own kind; this leads to focal patterns of both residence and sites of association, where prospective partners usually meet.

It was this study that led me to picture the various STD in the community as "propagating in small geodesic-shaped networks connected to larger networks in clusters that resemble syncytia formation with varying degrees of fusion between networks."[4] (Syncytia are clusters of cells that are fused together.) The central idea is that each STD is likely transmitted within different, definable, and well bounded populations, and that each of these specific populations, which maintained a specific STD in the community, was made up of persons who did not sexually mix very often with members of the other at-risk populations. It may be easier to visualize the community distribution of different STD in a community as resembling (say) a large soap bubble with other bubbles of varying sizes attached to its surface in one glob. The flat, two-dimensional graph below helps illustrate this concept. Wallace referred to these as "Potterat structures"[5-6] "viewing them as fundamental ecologic units of STD transmission" and "propose[d] mathematically that transmission occurs on the structures' surface in a one-dimensional 'travelling wave' fashion."[4-6]

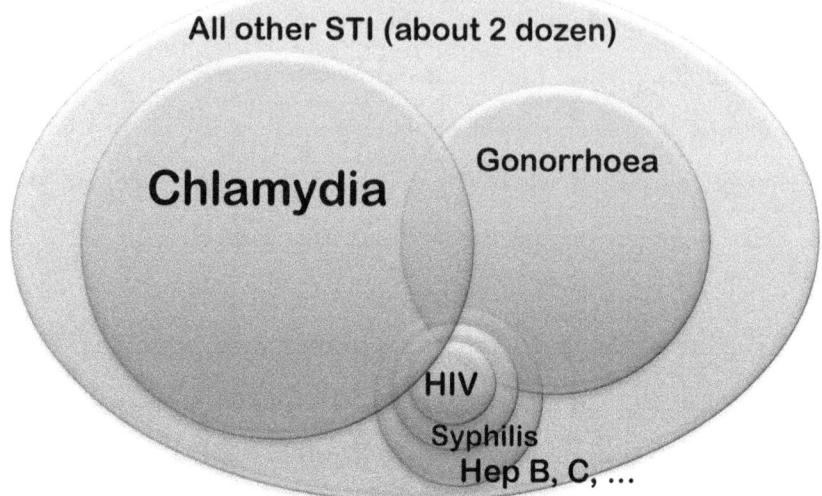

Figure 2.   Typical community case distribution of the many
             STI in bounded "Potterat Structures"

Based on illustration in our article in *Today's Life Science*.[4]
Designs by Steve Muth, October 1992 and October 2015.

Importantly, to summarize, this study demonstrated once more the power of contact tracing to elucidate an STD's epidemiologic patterns; this time, it was chlamydia's turn.

The Times, They Are A-Changin':[7] The influence of media reports

The emergence of chlamydia control in mid-1987 Colorado Springs occurred in context of relentless media reports and burgeoning anxiety in the general population about the AIDS threat to heterosexuals. A previous media campaign, which started in the late 1970s and focused on the "incurable STD" genital herpes, had already served to diminish the adventurism that had so often characterized young people's sex lives in the 1960s and 1970s. By the mid-1980s not only HIV, but also gonorrhea and syphilis incidence rates were waning, with the populations most susceptible to behavior change altering the demographics of STD populations. Young whites, straight and gay, were decreasingly represented in current STD/HIV acquisition, while young non-white representation was proportionally increasing. Susceptible populations may be viewed as layers of an onion; the layers containing those most susceptible to self-defense messages drop out of the risk pool first, followed later by layers containing those who take a bit more persuasion to join the ranks observing safer sex, to the layers containing those in chronic denial or who are unconcerned ("If God wants me to have this shit, there isn't much I can do about it"). In Chapter 6 we will see that sexual network structure influences STD risk over and above sexual behavior alone, so that it is possible for two different populations with similar sexual behavior attributes to experience very different prevalences of STD in their communities.[8] In any case, over time, it is the inner core layers that maintain STD reservoirs.[4]

We witnessed this evolution, initially with gonorrhea, because it was a reportable STD and because there were sufficient cases. For example, prior to the herpes scare years, say in 1975, the percentage of gonorrhea cases in blacks in Colorado Springs was about 30%; by 1982—during the herpes scare and before AIDS reports in heterosexuals—it was 53%.[9] During the heterosexual AIDS scare years, reported gonorrhea cases diminished from 1530 in 1985 to 861 in 1989, a 44% decline; importantly, the proportion accounted for by blacks increased from 49% to 62%.[10]

As for chlamydia, a similar evolution occurred: in 1988, 61% of public clinics cases were reported in whites, compared to 37% a dozen years later; the proportion in blacks doubled, from 20% in 1988 to 40% in 1999; as for Hispanics, their proportion remained stable at 19% (the other 3% comprised non-white "Other").[11]

Landmark studies in chlamydia transmission dynamics

By mid-1995 we switched to a new generation of chlamydia test based on polymerase chain-reaction (PCR) technology; not only was this new test considerably more accurate than our previously used tests, but we could now afford it. Universal, rather than targeted, use of this test in our clinics was made possible by our health department director's decision to allocate the required extra funds—this at a time when competition for adequate funding in any department was a considerable struggle.

The first chlamydia epidemiologic investigation using this exceptionally accurate test on a broad basis spanned the year 1 July 1996 to 30 June 1997. This study is another classic example of the power of contact tracing data to illuminate and validate crucial aspects of STD transmission dynamics. By 1996, chlamydia infection had been a reportable disease in Colorado for 4 years; we were hence able to assure contact interviewing of all reported cases in Colorado Springs— from the private, quasi-private, and military sectors—not simply those diagnosed in our public clinics. Of the 1,309 chlamydia cases reported during this 12-month period, we were able to interview 86%, yielding 2,409 contacts.[12] These data provided the opportunity to examine the reproductive rate of different chlamydia diagnostic categories by sex and by symptoms; we demonstrated that only one category, men with non-symptomatic urethral infection, came close (0.94) to exceeding the basic reproductive rate (> 1.0) required to maintain the disease in the community. All other categories hovered around 0.5. Since we had already demonstrated with gonorrhea contact tracing a dozen years earlier[13] that only men with non-symptomatic urethral gonorrhea had a reproductive rate greater than 1 (1.3 to be exact), the combined message from these studies was that men with non-symptomatic urethral chlamydia or gonorrhea infection should be accorded high intervention priority in control efforts. Remarkably, in both studies the overall reproductive rate hovered around 0.5, meaning that absent constant reintroduction of infection from outside our jurisdiction, each STD should soon die out in Colorado Springs. Although the chlamydia study was more comprehensive—because it included reproductive rate data on both men and women whereas the gonorrhea study included only heterosexual men—in both was the connection between reproductive rate and epidemic phase empirically demonstrated for the first time. (The 5 epidemic phases for STD spread are: introduction of a specific STD, establishment, growth, maintenance, and decline).

Colorado Springs's chlamydia incidence was indeed declining during this period, from about 300 cases per 100,000 during 1988 to about 200 per 100,000 by the end of 1997, a 33% decline. Although a good part of the decline may be attributed to augmented screening of susceptible women during this 10-year period, most of it was associated with expanded contact tracing, as shown in the following Figure.[12]

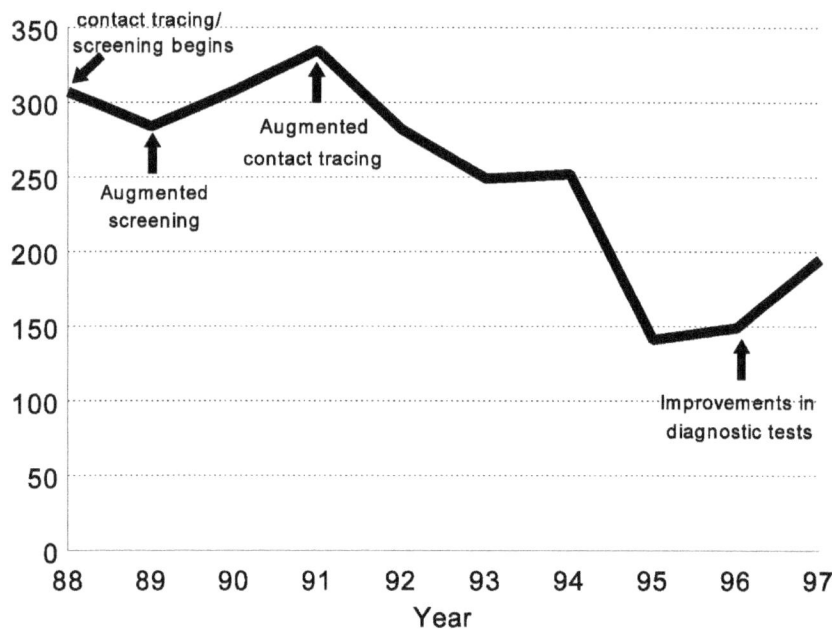

Figure 3: Reported chlamydia cases in Colorado Springs, 1988–1997, and impact of interventions (screening, contact tracing, and use of improved diagnostic tests)

Y-axis: cases per 100,000 population. X-axis: year of reports

Reprinted, with permission, from our article in the
American Journal of Epidemiology[12]—Graphic by Steve Muth.

Of special importance in this chlamydia study was demonstration, also for the first time, of the crucial role played by sexual partner concurrency in STD transmission.[12] Cases with concurrent, as opposed to serial, sexual partners were much more likely to be successful chlamydia transmitters than those cases who merely had multiple contacts. Although concurrency was indeed highly correlated with number of sexual partners, the odds of being a transmitter were twice as great for those whose multiple partnerships were concurrent. Demonstration that the effect of concurrency was not confounded by number of contacts was a signal achievement. And what gave this achievement special credibility was the type of evidence buttressing it. Our observations were derived from epidemiologic data that are as close to transmission events as can be obtained in public health investigation: on the ground contact tracing information.

Yet another notable result from this study was empiric delineation of chlamydia's infectious periods.[14] Because chlamydia infection seldom proclaims itself with genital symptoms, it was generally difficult for newly diagnosed patients to know how long they might have harbored the infection and, therefore, which non-current sexual partners to notify. Trying to develop a sense for how long a non-symptomatic patient of either sex might have been infectious could most reliably be estimated using quality contact tracing data. Although previously done for gonorrhea,[15-18] it had not yet been done for chlamydia. The available CDC recommendations at the time (1997) were based on limited and unpublished data.[19] Combining use of the now highly reliable PCR test with community-wide chlamydia contact tracing presented a singular opportunity to define infectious periods. Our results showed that the CDC recommendations, although based on soft data, were adequate; they could be expected to identify 88% of the infected contacts who were unaware of their infection. Unfortunately for the community, the 12% of infected, untreated contacts who would not be identified by the CDC algorithm were mostly non-symptomatic men whose chronic infection was shown to be of very long duration. These silently infected men, unlike silently infected women who were routinely being screened, were unlikely to have their infection intercepted; the data indicated that they formed the substrate for the entrenched reservoir of chlamydia in the community, echoing the same mechanism we noted for gonorrhea entrenchment in the late 1970s.[20] In both instances, because non-symptomatic men were not likely to be screened for either STD or, as we once again documented, not likely to be successfully referred to examination by their partners, active public health intervention was indicated.[21] Specifically, such an intervention needed to focus on eliciting and tracing the temporally distant male partners missed by the CDC algorithm.

In neither instance did publication of our data result in much more than lip service attention by public health authorities, in spite of the fact that our data validated mathematical and decision-analysis models.[22-24] Screening of high-risk men remained under-advocated and, most importantly, unfunded. This was not surprising, if only because chlamydia control funding was living in the shadow of a giant competitor: AIDS.[1]

It is ironic that official CDC recommendations for the control of STD emphasize the importance of evidence-based information and at the same time inexplicably ignore quality empiric evidence such as that meticulously collected during the last quarter of the 20th century in Colorado Springs.[21] These studies were most often published in respected medical and public health journals; they clearly provided compelling evidence for the importance of identifying and treating men with non-symptomatic urethral gonorrhea or chlamydia. In the official, recent guidelines for management of STD/HIV contacts, not only are non-symptomatic men not mentioned but, bafflingly, the limelight is placed on *symptomatic* patients;[25, p. 17] none of our key papers supporting the importance of silently infected non-symptomatic men in community disease entrenchment is cited in their voluminous references. Our papers were notable and should have carried weight, because they provided strong and consistent empiric evidence of a rare commodity in the STD control literature: evidence of *positive impact* on the disease burden. The CDC oversight is baffling not only because I was one of the outside consultants for these recommendations and, indeed, had pointed out these epidemiologic realities during our deliberations, but also because 3 years before I had specifically taken CDC researchers to task in a mainstream STD journal[21] for not having done their homework in the gonorrhea and chlamydia contact tracing literature; this specific publication listed all the key overlooked papers.[21] Moreover, the CDC ignored results of our empiric efforts to improve STD/HIV contact interviewing techniques[26] and failed to recommend these (cost-free) improvements in empirically-validated techniques[26–29] despite multiple presentations to CDC staff by principal investigator (and colleague) Dr. Devon Brewer.

It is disappointing that our painstakingly collected evidence consistently fell on deaf ears, perhaps because these ears tended to be those of clinicians, whose professional paradigm is disease *acquisition-* (rather than disease *transmission-*) oriented. Or perhaps it's because health bureaucracies make decisions by committee—which implies emphasis on consensus building—rather than by individuals whose focus is on assessing the availability and quality of the evidence.

Augmenting the value of contact tracing data through network analysis

Our last chlamydia contact tracing study turned out to be the icing on the STD epidemiology cake. Although it appears that we saved the best part for last, this was not intentional. In the mid-1990s, the CDC's Wasserheit and Aral proposed that the efficacy and efficiency of STD public health interventions might be enhanced were these interventions epidemic-phase-specific.[30] The crucial problem was diagnosis: it was said that phase-appropriate interventions would depend on reliable assessment of current STD epidemic phase in a given community. Accurate assessment of whether an STD's incidence was growing, stable, or declining was fraught with difficulty, because assessment of the magnitude and direction of STD transmission customarily relied on potentially flawed evidence. This traditional evidence was known to have many artifacts: it relied on secular trend analysis of reported STD cases or of surrogate markers (for example, visits to emergency rooms or private doctors for genital symptoms complaints). Such data had serious shortcomings stemming from the reliability of diagnostic tests used; from the completeness of their use at the clinical or population level; from the vagaries of case definition; from the consistency of case reporting; and to changes in at-risk populations (for example, large scale rotations of locally stationed servicemen) or in interventions (for example, fluctuating intensity of STD contact tracing and screening initiatives). Were these obstacles surmountable and, if so, how?

During the decade preceding publication of the Wasserheit-Aral paper,[30] our STD/HIV control program had implemented—and analyzed data from—the first empiric study of the influence of the conformation of sexual and drug networks on STD/HIV transmission. This endeavor, prompted by the CDC's interest in studying the susceptibility of high-risk heterosexuals to HIV acquisition and transmission, concluded that the conformation of risk networks had a profound influence on providing pathways for STD/HIV diffusion or on presenting constraints to diffusion. Dubbed CDC Project 90, details of this investigation and its findings form the subject of Chapter 6. In brief for now, the architect of Project 90, the sociologist Alden Klovdahl, introduced us to a paradigm imported from his professional discipline, network analysis.[31] By the time we initiated the long-term chlamydia contact tracing initiative in 1996 we were familiar with the power of network analysis to augment the value of STD/HIV contact tracing data through its ability to connect case-contact pairs at both the micro- and macro-levels. Although we did not intend or design the study to relate contact tracing data to epidemic phase we decided, upon completion of data collection at the end of 1999, to analyze these data using network analysis. Our interest was programmatic: to explore and explain the fluctuating trend in chlamydia reported cases noted during the study interval (1996–1999), as described below.

Our original intention was to measure the impact of saturation contact tracing on chlamydia incidence—a repeat performance from our gonorrhea epidemic days (Chapter 2), as it were, but with a different STD. The chlamydia contact tracing initiatives of the late 1980s through the 1990s echoed the gonorrhea contact tracing initiatives of the late 1970s through the early 1980s in Colorado Springs. With gonorrhea, we had started with focal contact tracing on selected populations and then followed, once resources were available, with saturation contact tracing, as described in Chapter 2. This time, we followed the focal chlamydia contact tracing endeavor which characterized the first 8 years (1988 through 1995) with saturation efforts from 1996 through 1999. And just as each of the gonorrhea contact tracing initiatives occasioned substantial reductions in incidence between 1976 and 1982, each of the chlamydia contact tracing endeavors, focal and saturation, was associated with incidence decline. [12,21,32] More importantly for the long view, our late 1990s saturation contact tracing initiative occasioned the most comprehensive and detailed analysis of community chlamydia transmission ever reported, producing yet another landmark paper.[32]

To summarize the salient features of this study: all cases of chlamydia diagnosed in the Colorado Springs region were reported to our STD surveillance unit, as required by the state law passed in November 1991. Between January 1996 and December 1999, 6067 cases of chlamydia in adults were reported from the public (44%), military (30%), and private (26%) sectors. Three-quarters (4593) were interviewed for sexual partner information; they named 7365 contacts. Together, cases and their contacts comprised 9114 unique individuals. Network analysis of the connections between these nearly 10,000 individuals (in a community of 500,000) revealed network conformations highly suggestive of stable (conservatively) to declining (liberally) incidence.[32–33] Although during this 4-year period, reported cases per 100,000 increased from 255 in 1996 to 373 in 1999, converging evidence from multiple data sources clearly associated increasing case reports with gradual implementation of the extremely accurate chlamydia PCR test in our community, first in our health department clinics in mid-1996, followed 2 years later in military clinics, and more sporadically during this interval in private doctor practices. We labeled it a "phony" epidemic,[32] for it was so evidently an artifact of testing and enhanced contact tracing: we had, starting in 1996, increased contact interviewing of chlamydia cases by 38%, and increased partner tracing by 70%, compared to the previous 8 years. Important evidence to support true incidence decline consisted of the multiple changes in reasons for case detection for both men and women, which suggested shifts from passive to active case detection and, among other reasons, the 20% decline in symptoms of pelvic inflammatory disease in our clinics. Again the detailed evidence presented in that paper echoes that recorded to show that the declines in gonorrhea incidence of the 1976–1982 periods were genuine and related to our interventions, particularly contact tracing.

In addition, we presented detailed descriptions of the geographic and demographic attributes of members of the connected components likeliest to be responsible for perpetuating chlamydia transmission in Colorado Springs. In particular, specific sexual mixing patterns, which had previously been associated with STD core group membership, were now examined in context of the (few, see below) well-connected components we had, along with other transmission-associated diagnostic characteristics (for example, recent repeaters and dually-infected people). Network analysis revealed why these core group members were such important actors in transmission.

As for epidemic phase, analysis of network configurations during the 4-year study interval revealed a structural environment supportive of low chlamydia propagation. This was confirmed in a comparison of contemporaneous network configurations of chlamydia cases in Manitoba, Canada.[33] These network analyses required specialized skills and creation of computer routines (especially name matching routines) that were not available commercially—tasks brilliantly accomplished, via dogged determination and felicitous algorithmic insights, by our information systems manager, Steve Muth. Although there were some relatively large connected components, the vast majority of connected individuals resided in small components: 2122 (79%) of the total 2701 separate components hosted only 2 or 3 people each, and 2625 (97%) consisted of 9 or fewer connected people. This structural configuration did not change during the 4-year interval. This suggested an anemic transmission environment, a conclusion that was supported by almost all of the study data we had collected. Network cohesion, which is strongly predictive of STD transmission intensity was minimal. Importantly we showed that determination of epidemic phase can be quickly assessed using a few months of contact tracing data filtered through network analysis; this procedure is likely to be much quicker than waiting months or years to discern secular trends. Accurate assessment of epidemic phase and its associated network structure can also provide the rationale for emphasizing one intervention over another. For example, in an environment essentially composed of fragmented structures, targeted screening for chlamydia may be more effective than contact tracing, whereas in an environment containing densely connected components, contact tracing may be the superior way to fragment transmission pathways and thus interrupt transmissions.

In sum, this investigation provided persuasive evidence for the usefulness of applying network analysis to contact tracing data to accurately gauge epidemic phase. Network tools were glaringly illuminating; they not only reliably detailed community transmission dynamics, but also choreographed its epidemic phase. A final bonus of application of network analysis to contact tracing data is ease of demonstrating impact on disease incidence, the Holy Grail of STD control endeavors. The marriage of on-the-ground contact tracing data—in the capable hands of Helen Zimmerman-Rogers—with network tools—in the capable hands of Steve Muth —constitutes one of the truly important descriptive and analytic developments in STD/HIV epidemiology in the last half-century.

FIVE

PROSTITUTION & STD/HIV CONTROL

Part 1. Prostitute women: the supply side

Prostitution and venereal disease: a time-honored connection

In the popular mind, the link between venereal disease and prostitution is of hoary antiquity. During the 1970s, this link was in our professional mind as well. And for good reason. In the late 1960s, the American Social Health Association had conducted an ethnographic survey in Colorado Springs that suggested high levels of venereal infections in prostitutes, while contact interviews with infected men suggested that prostitutes were probably responsible, directly or indirectly, for most local gonorrhea transmission, principally through their sexual liaisons with U.S. servicemen.[1]

As previously described (Chapter 2), we implemented the Health Hold Order system in 1970 to pressure prostitutes into periodic examination for the two reportable venereal infections: gonorrhea and syphilis.[1–2] Colorado communicable disease statutes (CRS 25-4-404) not only mandated that "health officers investigate sources of infections of venereal disease" but—and this may surprise the reader—"to cooperate with the proper officials whose duty it is to enforce laws directed against prostitution…" Cooperation with the police to suppress prostitution made public health officers uncomfortable; we chose to suppress venereal disease transmission instead. For the next 30 years, cooperation with the police was a one-way street: they provided access to their prostitution surveillance and arrest records, while medical confidentiality prevented us from revealing our information. The police understood our position and (reluctantly) acquiesced.

To nurture cooperation between prostitutes and our VD control program, we used both carrot and stick. We met them on their own turf, frequently visiting the stroll (soliciting areas) to encourage them to visit our VD Clinic monthly. Once in clinic, we treated them with dignity and accorded them rapid service. Their charts were color-coded so that staff members knew who needed speedy service—not fair to the other patients, but nobody was under the illusion that life was fair. That was the carrot. The stick consisted of vigorous, consistent application of the Health Hold Order, where arrested prostitutes were not released from jail until tested for venereal diseases. Not only did we rely on a climate of goodwill to interrupt VD transmission but, in the process, learned so much about them and their lives that our on-the-ground ethnographic approach spawned unexpected insights and useful data which would, over a quarter century, be reported in the scholarly literature.

An example of our outreach efforts on the stroll was published in the CDC's *Morbidity and Mortality Weekly Report*.[3] We offered risk reduction advice specifically tailored for (the often injecting drug using) street prostitutes and distributed free condoms for both oral (dry, mint flavored), and below the belt (lubricated) sex, front or back. We counseled them about safer sexual and injecting drug use behaviors, encouraging them and their clients to visit our VD Clinic and enroll in our drug treatment programs. On average, one of us spent about an hour a day on the stroll, reaching half a dozen prostitutes and distributing about 300 condoms a week. These activities were associated with declines in positivity on syphilis, gonorrhea, and chlamydia tests obtained from Colorado Springs prostitutes, though corroborating evidence to link positivity declines with condom distribution was regrettably not collected.[1,3]

Impact of contact tracing and use of the Health Hold system on the STD burden

As provided in detail elsewhere,[1-4] conscientious application of both the Health Hold Order and, especially, of contact tracing served to dramatically reduce the STD burden in Colorado Springs during the last 3 decades of the 20th century. The Health Hold system itself was discontinued after a quarter-century, because by the 1990s, venereal infections were declining rapidly in examined prostitutes. Although of the virtually 5,000 examinations performed between June 1970 and December 1994 (the Health Hold period), 16.5% yielded positive gonorrhea tests overall; the annual percentage declined in stepwise fashion from a high of 31% in the early 1970s to about 13% between 1976 and 1990, to 6% in the early 1990s, to 1.6% during the second half of the 1990s. Chlamydia positivity declined as well, but not as steeply: from 12% in 1988 (first full year of testing) to 5.4% at the end of both 1994 and the rest of the 1990s. In brief, about 1% of the community's gonorrhea burden, and 0.5% of chlamydia cases, were diagnosed in prostitute women during the second half of the 1990s, testifying to their much diminished role in STD transmission in Colorado Springs compared to their significant contributions in earlier periods, starting in the late 1960s.

Testing for HIV infection was not mandatory, yet virtually all (732 of 768, or 95%) women with histories of prostitution were voluntarily tested since availability of the test in mid-1985 through 1999; 28 (3.8%) had positive tests. At least 24 of the 28 HIV-infected prostitutes provided a history of injecting drug use and 4 didn't, though we suspected that at least 2 of the latter were not forthcoming about their real risk factors.[5]

Prostitutes and ethnographic observations:
insights and longitudinal data

At a minimum, prostitutes tolerated (more likely, accepted) us on their turf and on the margins of their personal lives. From this privileged position, we were able to "observe a lot by watching" during 3 decades, as Yogi Berra memorably said. My first epiphany about prostitute women occurred as a consequence of my colleague Lynanne Phillips outlining the lives of women she was contact-interviewing for our study of the antecedents of gonococcal pelvic inflammation.[6–7] These women's biographies seemed to echo the lives of prostitutes I was meeting on the stroll and in the VD clinic. If this biographical correspondence was shown to be real, then what determined entry into prostitution could not simply be sociology—the conventional explanatory model, which usually blamed various adverse socio-familial factors.[8] In brief, there simply had to be determining psychological or characterological factors. As I wrote later, "...social factors may set the stage for prostitution, but the script to become a prostitute may be written by psychological factors".[9]

On becoming a prostitute (Part I: 1976):
an exploratory case-comparison study

And so, with the help of CDC sociologist Dr. Bill Darrow, we structured a small exploratory study for clues about women's entry into prostitution. Though conducted during 1976, results were not made public until 3 years later, at a scientific meeting in Boston, and not published until virtually a decade after completion of data collection.[8] This glacial pace was my fault: I had neither the scientific training, familiarity with the scholarly prostitution literature, nor the necessary tools to analyze the data, while the expert, Dr. Darrow, had too many competing demands for his time and analytic energies. (Dr. Darrow was, as part of the original CDC Task Force on AIDS, at the forefront of efforts to elucidate this deadly new syndrome during 1981–1982.)

In this exploratory study, we compared life experiences of 14 of the 90 street prostitutes observed during 1976 with those of 15 promiscuous women we periodically cared for in our VD Clinic. (Of 15 prostitutes approached one refused our offer; all comparisons approached agreed to participate.) Because this was a pilot investigation, no attempt was made to obtain a random sample for either street prostitutes or their non-prostitute comparisons. Probed topics included: childhood, adolescent, and adult experiences regarding: family life; religious upbringing; schooling; health; finances; social, romantic, and sexual activities; personal crises and coping mechanisms. Most of the characteristics and experiences reported by the 14 prostitutes mirrored those reported by the promiscuous non-prostitute women. As for differences, prostitutes tended to be first-born children; more interested in completing school than the comparison women; and less likely to shun sexual partners of different ethnicities. Many of the non-prostitutes had been exposed to other women who engaged in prostitution but chose different ways of solving their financial and other problems. Indeed, aversion to accepting money for sex was the most important reason given by the promiscuous non-prostitutes for not engaging in prostitution; they equated sex with their own pleasure, not someone else's.

At the time of our pilot investigation, very few studies exploring risk factors for entry into prostitution had used control groups of non-prostitute women. Of the 3 we had found in the literature,[10–12] each reported similar results: few if any differences between prostitutes and control women were noted. Their reports, then, along with ours, raised serious questions about the validity of the conventional "environmental factors are at fault" model. However, much stronger support for the view that psychological factors may be primary in the causal path to prostitution had to await implementation of an empiric study we conducted in Colorado Springs a decade and a half later and which also, for reasons similar to those presented above, took 6 years post data collection to appear in print.[9] But it was worth the long incubation, for publication of our data won the Hugo Beigel Award for best article published in the *Journal of Sex Research* in 1998.

On becoming a prostitute (Part II: 1990–1992): the chronology of sexual and drug abuse milestones

With the arrival of AIDS came burgeoning interest in female prostitution and its role in transmission of this deadly virus in heterosexual populations. As previously described (See Chapter 3), we had collaborated with the CDC study which aimed to elucidate HIV prevalence and associated risk factors in U.S. prostitute women.[13–16] At least 2 other issues interested the public health establishment: obtaining a robust estimate of the prostitute population in America, and elucidating factors influencing entry into prostitution. The former would provide CDC a sense for how large the at-risk population was, while the latter could inform potentially effective interventions aimed at minimizing adverse sexual and drug abuse outcomes. Our program was in a position to obtain data to help answer both queries. A little later, I describe our empirically derived prostitute population estimates for both Colorado Springs and for the nation. Presently I describe our attempt to find clues about why women enter prostitution by exploring some antecedents to entry. Specifically, we focus on describing the sequence, timing, and prevalence of sexual and drug abuse events in the lives of prostitute women, comparing findings to those of non-prostitute women.

Prostitution has a long past, but a short history.[9] (This was my paraphrase of Ebbinghaus's "Psychology has a long past, but a short history".) In my view, this is because gathering reliable information from representative samples of prostitutes is fraught with difficulty; prostitute populations tend to be defensive, elusive, fluid, and not easily accessed by researchers. In Colorado Springs, our constant and trusted association with prostitutes since 1970 provided an opportunity to collect data from the entire population, not just from some convenience samples. It was our intent that the data we planned to collect would be of use, perhaps pointing the way to interventions that could reduce the twin public health burdens of prostitution: substance abuse and STD/HIV transmission. At the very least, it was hoped that findings would challenge the widely circulating pulp fiction versions of prostitution entry: that it was women who were sexually abused in childhood who were later seduced into prostitution by getting them hooked on street drugs.

Accordingly, between August 1990 and December 1992 we surveyed as many current and former prostitutes we knew in Colorado Springs. As has been true for all of our prostitution queries (except Project 90; see Chapter 6) this endeavor was unfunded; it was bonus work, meaning that finding out answers was its own reward. The survey instrument consisted of 9 short questions and was administered to current prostitutes (141 of 158 [90%] participated); former prostitutes (100 of 317 in our records were located, of whom 96% consented); and comparison women (407 of 475 [86%] who were eligible were interviewed). This represented a very high level of acceptance: only 13 prostitutes (5%) and 10 comparisons (2.4%) actually *refused* participation; failure to enroll other eligible prostitutes were administrative failures on our part.

Survey questions were aimed at delineating milestone events suspected of influencing entry into prostitution: age at first penile penetration anywhere in the body (with or without consent); age at first consensual sex and at first *regular* consensual sex; age at first (non-injectable) street drug use and at first *regular* street drug (exclusive of alcohol) use; age at first injectable street drug use and age at first *regular* injecting drug use; age at first prostitution and at first *regular* prostitution.[9]

In brief, here are the important results. Although a greater proportion of prostitutes (32%) reported penile penetration before age 11 compared to non-prostitute women (13%), the really striking difference between these two groups was drug abuse: 86% of prostitutes reported

111

regular street drug use versus 23% for comparison women. Moreover, one half of prostitutes (60% of former, and 43% of current, prostitutes) had ever injected street drugs versus 4% in comparisons. Notably, two-thirds of prostitutes had used illicit drugs *before* entering prostitution and three-quarters who had ever *injected* street drugs reported doing so *before* entering prostitution. An association between sexual activity and drug abuse was also noted in our sample of non-prostitute women; those who reported regular street drug use were significantly more sexually active than those who were not—an average of 4.0 sexual partners in the previous 12 months vs. 2.7 for non-drug users, and 14.7 lifetime partners compared to 10.6 for non-drug users.

The few previously published studies[17-19] reporting a relationship between initiation of street drug use and prostitution entry reached a similar conclusion: drug abuse usually precedes entry into the life. What made ours more definitive was that our data, unlike those previously available, were derived not from convenience samples, but from the population itself *and* were compared to data from matched controls. In addition, the validity of our data was assessed. Skeptics usually assume that prostitutes are more likely to lie on surveys than non-prostitute women. We therefore decided to re-administer the 9-question survey to prostitutes about a year later; we were able to locate nearly two-fifths (92/237) of the prostitutes—mostly those who were residents rather than just passing through. Survey concordance was high: 43% of resurveyed prostitutes gave identical answers; 70% provided answers that were within a year of the original response; and 84% provided answers within 2 years of the original response.[9]

Establishing a temporal link between drug abuse and prostitution entry with reliable data was important, because drug abuse can be viewed as a powerful lever to infer reasons for entry. In the psychiatric literature, substance abuse has been shown to be a marker of psychological problems and mental illness. (Drug use is presumably used by distressed patients to self-medicate.) Hence if, as we have convincingly shown, drug abuse precedes entry, this sets the stage for further development of theory that can link specific psychological factors in the causal pathway to prostitution: psychological distress leads to substance abuse, and specific psychological configurations may facilitate entry into the life. Be that as it may, from earliest days, my sense from the literature was that the dominant narrative viewed prostitutes as victims of external circumstances, particularly of abusive environments. Our original report[8] and subsequent studies from a few other researchers[20–21] suggested that psychological factors may well be of primary importance in the decision to enter prostitution. Hence exploring internal factors should assume greater attention on the part of researchers than simply focusing on external ones. To borrow from the infectious disease literature, being successfully "infected" requires both exposure and susceptibility. The present study reinforced, with much stronger data, our original conclusion[8] that while environmental factors might set the stage for prostitution (exposure) the script to become a prostitute is most likely written by specific psychological factors (susceptibility).

While our two studies suggested, along with those of a few others, that psychological or characterological factors were likely to play a dominant role, precisely which profiles these were eluded us until our colleague Dr. Stuart Brody, a trained clinical psychologist, offered to review the prostitution literature and our previous work to try to distill these profiles. His review in the early 2000s indicated that antisocial personality disorder, along with borderline personality disorder, were the principal psychopathological characteristics of street prostitutes[22] (but not of call girls). For example, of the 7 criteria listed for Antisocial Personality Disorder, it was likely that the minimum requirement of 3 criteria to support this diagnosis would commonly be met by our street prostitutes. The criteria: 1) failure to conform to social norms with respect to lawful behaviors, as indicated by repeatedly performing acts that are grounds for arrest; 2) deceitfulness (e.g., use of multiple aliases; feigning erotic response during sex); 3) impulsiveness; 4) aggressiveness, as manifested by assaults (prostitutes as perpetrators); 5) reckless disregard for safety of self or others (e.g., entering potentially dangerous places for sex with strangers); 6) consistent irresponsibility (e.g., failure to pay taxes for their work; frequent allegations of child neglect by social services); 7) lack of remorse. Dr. Brody's review also corroborated our finding, based on use of the CES-D (Center for Epidemiologic Studies Depression Scale) test on a small convenience sample, that clinical depression was common among prostitute women.[23] He also found that reports of dissociative disorders, posttraumatic stress disorder (PTSD), and so-called Cluster A (paranoid, schizoid) personality disorders were common in the literature on prostitute women.[22]

In brief, Brody's review made it apparent that (ironically) lack of appreciation for sexual intercourse; antisocial and/or borderline personality disorders; clinical depression; and predisposition to disassociation and PTSD, were salient features of street prostitutes' psychological landscapes. Notably, this view can persuasively explain why *so few* women enter prostitution, despite the exciting lures of sexual adventurism and easy money. This composite profile resonates with my impressionistic observations of street prostitute women during my three decades on the stroll.

No summary of prostitute women's psychological landscapes should omit discussion of some of its untoward and discouraging consequences. We implemented a small pilot project in the early 1990s; during the 19 months between September 1993 and March 1995, we recruited 17 prostitutes, and 50 comparison women at risk to enter prostitution, to assess their receptivity for community services that could provide alternatives to prostitution.[23] Participants were interviewed at baseline and again 6 and 12 months after our offer of case management services. A dedicated, sympathetic, and experienced public health nurse (once again Lynanne Plummer-Phillips) offered emotional support, personalized referrals, and assistance in reducing

115

bureaucratic and financial obstacles. Referrals focused on socio-economic, medical, mental health, and rehabilitative services.

Participants were highly selective about acceptance: follow-through for rehabilitative services was low, despite sustained coaching and encouragement. The success rate was only 9% for mental health, 0% for substance abuse, and 44% for educational, services. In addition, 81% of participants were classified as depressed. We hypothesized that these discouraging results were linked to psychological problems, foremost among them depression.[23] You can lead a horse to water...

Estimating the prevalence and career longevity
of prostitute women (1988)

In the early 1980s the emergence of HIV, which can be transmitted both sexually and by contaminated needles, naturally generated interest on the part of the public health establishment because of the potential contribution to HIV transmission by prostitutes. Not only were they by definition sexually active, but about half of prostitutes were reportedly injecting street drugs. Hence, developing a sense for the prevalence, career longevity, and prevalence of risky behaviors of prostitutes was deemed a priority by the National Research Council in the late 1980s.[24] In thinking about this national request, it occurred to me that given our long and mutually trusted association with prostitutes, and given our relatively easy access to them should we want to survey them, our program could perhaps make a useful contribution. The key to my decision to help was knowing that, for two decades, we had kept meticulous records of visits to our VD Clinic by various kinds of (street-, hotel-, massage parlor-based) prostitutes and that we had compared publicly available lists of local prostitution arrests by the police with our prostitute list every few years. Even more important was availability of resources to consolidate our VD Clinic chart- and logbooks-based information by entering twenty years of data into our newly purchased microcomputer (our Program's first, in late 1987! See Appendix 1) to attempt an estimate. (We christened our computer prostitution database "Lady Jane" to honor D.H. Lawrence's heroine Lady Chatterley's private parts.) We had recently received funding from the CDC to conduct Project 90. These monies not only brought back Donald Woodhouse, after a 5-year detour to attend Law School and establish a private practice, but enabled us to hire a brilliant techie, Steve Muth. None of the impressive estimates we were able to distill from our available records would have been possible without their help.

Once the laborious task of data entry was completed and we were able to examine data frequencies, we immediately noted the essentially regular annual distribution of prostitutes visits during the nearly two decades from 1970 through 1988; although the range was a bit wide (from a low of 54 in 1974 to a high of 164 in 1977), the average was usually about 100 (Mean=98; median=94).[25] That was encouraging, for wild fluctuations in numbers would likely have undermined our confidence in any attempt to derive a national estimate. But prostitutes captured by our system were not all equal: some, we knew, had only appeared on our radar screen for a brief period, while others for a long time. Accordingly, I decided to label each prostitute by the amount of time she had apparently stayed in Colorado Springs: 1) <u>evanescent prostitutes</u> had offered their services for a short period, usually around military paydays (bi-weekly) and then resumed soliciting on their customary circuit; 2) <u>short-term prostitutes</u> may have intended to stay but were discouraged because of poor marketplace conditions, personal preference, or police pressure—in any year, they were present for many weeks to many months; 3) <u>long-term prostitutes</u> usually solicited for several years, even if not continuously. To derive a reasonably accurate quantitative sense of the supply side of prostitution, I arbitrarily assigned an annual weight to each member of each category: 0.1 for evanescent prostitutes, because they were seldom present for more than 30–40 days in a year; 0.5 for short-termers, because they were typically seen over a period of several months during the year; and 1.0 for long-termers, because they were observed locally almost all year. (The year before, I had used a similar weighting scheme to estimate the contribution to local gonorrhea transmission by each kind of contact featured in STD contact interviews.[26]) This weighting scheme, when applied to our prostitutes, generated an estimate of the number of "full-time equivalent" prostitutes (FTEP) in our database, thereby reducing the probability of overestimating the "true" number of prostitutes nationally. This scheme produced a similar secular trend for these two decades; again, although the range was wide (36.7–109.4 FTEPs), the average was nearly 70 (Mean=69.3; Median=67.7) with no wild fluctuations. This stable level was also promising for our attempt to derive a valid national estimate using our historical data: year after year, we experienced a similar distribution of evanescent, short-term, and long-term prostitutes. When we grafted our local FTEP data to the annual U.S. general population estimates for the interval 1970–1988, we found similar stability in the number of FTEPs per 100,000 population: although the range was a bit wide (38,500–100,300 FTEPs nationally), the average was about 60,000 (Mean=62,600; Median=56,300).[25]

To compensate for any health department shortfall in observation during this nearly two decade period, I decided to use a mathematical formula I had recently been introduced to by reading an article in the journal *Science*. [27] This formula was manna from heaven, coming at precisely the right time. A "capture-recapture" method, it was designed to estimate the size of elusive populations. To estimate completeness of our prostitute counts, we needed to enter, into this formula, the number of prostitute women observed by the police, multiplied by the number observed by our health department, divided by the number of prostitutes observed in common by both sources during a specified interval and the product was the "true" estimate. The long and the short of it was that our health department database contained an estimated 79% of the true total in Colorado Springs. We thus retrofitted this percentage to infer a current national estimate. The result? There were about 77,500 prostitutes (52,700 FTEPs) in the U.S. during 1988. Averaged over the previous nine years—the AIDS era—

we obtained a national estimate of 84,000 prostitutes (59,000 FTEPs) per year. Since FTEP data are less likely to count women from different areas multiple times, this FTEP estimate probably approximated reality better than the unadjusted number. Lastly, we were able to derive, from our prostitution surveillance data, a robust estimate of duration of prostitution: street prostitutes engaged in prostitution for an average of 4 (Median) to 5 (Mean) years, with a Range of 2–22 years.[25] Our data therefore seriously undermined the adage that "once a prostitute, always a prostitute".

Extrapolating the number of prostitute women working in the United States by using data from a single community in Middle America would be destined to invite much skepticism, if not derision, unless I could find supportive data. Such data would have to indicate that ours may be typical enough to represent the national mean. I used gonorrhea rates as a starting point: the national gonorrhea rate per 100,000 population at the time (1980–1987) was 388; ours was virtually identical: 394. I also argued that Colorado Springs had prostitution-market place characteristics of both small (total population) and large (because of the military) communities. In addition, I used results from a then recent probability sample of U.S. adults[28] who were surveyed about the number of sexual partners they had had during the previous 12 months. None of the women in the high-risk (18–44) years for prostitution reported any partnership for payment. This observation supported our apparently low estimate of the number of prostitutes in the U.S. (At the time, most estimates—"guesstimates", really—placed the numbers of U.S. prostitutes in the 200,000–500,000 range.) Importantly, our "low" estimate was in reasonable accord with the (probably conservative) FBI data showing that, between 1970 and 1987, a mean of 55,366 women (Median=57,890) were annually arrested for prostitution offenses in the United States. In any event, our work showed that the prostitute burden in the U.S. was not likely to be as large as suggested by the empirically unsupported numbers spawned by wild guesses. That, in itself, was a comforting contribution to the public health literature.

Mortality in prostitute women

Our long-term association with prostitutes in Colorado Springs and completeness of our observation records also presented an opportunity to rigorously assess some of prostitution's untoward outcomes, specifically premature mortality. Anecdotal information had long made us aware of the risk of premature death in such women. For example, we had previously reported that, among 89 practicing prostitutes observed during 1976, four had died, three by homicide and one by drug overdose.[2] Five-year mortality in a group of (prostitute or not) women of this size and age structure would be 1.2 deaths; these deaths among our prostitutes had occurred in one year.

Published data on prostitute mortality were sparse. Other than the brief report mentioned in the previous paragraph[2], only one other graced the literature.[29] It was a study of health and safety hazards among prostitutes covering a nine-year period in London. No prior research had measured mortality in such women during a long period or had verified death and cause of death using official records. I wondered what it would take to produce an estimate using our prostitution records. My colleague Steve Muth, who had created the prostitution databases, told me that there was a free mortality database on the World Wide Web, the Social Security Death Index (SSDI), which listed decedents with social security numbers for whom survivor claims had been processed. "Free" suited our budget constraints perfectly. And so Steve and I, when time permitted, looked for confirmed deaths among our current and former prostitutes (1969 women between the years 1967 and 1999), thirty percent of whom had provided multiple names over time. This first step suggested that there indeed had been many deaths; regrettably, the SSDI database did not provide information on sex, race/ethnicity, birth name (for women), or place and cause of death. The relative insensitivity and shortcomings of the SSDI database compared to the official—and expensive—National Death Index (NDI) put us in the position of having to fish for funds to access the NDI. The NDI is maintained by the CDC and collects registered death information provided by state and territorial registries since 1979. It was Dr. Rothenberg who graciously provided the funds (approximately $8,600 from one of his grants) to pay for the NDI searches on our data.

Results in brief: of 1,969 prostitute women, 117 were confirmed dead by the end of 1997 in 26 different states (a testament to their peripatetic lifestyle). Based on our sometimes incomplete identifying information, an additional 26 were classified as possibly dead. Prostitute women were: 1) likelier to die by a factor of two compared to comparable women not known to be prostitutes; 2) six times more likely to die while actively engaged in prostitution compared to periods when they were not working; and 3) eighteen times more likely to be homicide victims while actively engaged in prostitution compared to women of similar age and race during the study interval.[5]

Few of the women died of natural causes, as would be expected for people whose average age at death was 34. (This datum tempted me to title the paper we eventually published: "The Half-Life of Prostitute Women". I was talked out of it.) Causes of death were, unsurprisingly, primarily attributable to violence and drug use: homicide (19%), drug abuse (18%), accidents (12%), alcohol-related (9%), and HIV (8%). HIV deaths occurred only among injecting drug users. Cancers, cardiovascular events, and various illnesses accounted for the remaining third of deaths.[5]

As of the time of this writing (Spring 2015) this study remains the only one of its kind in the literature—comprising a large longitudinal cohort of prostitutes whose inclusion is approximately *population-* (as opposed to *convenience sample-*) based, and whose mortality outcomes and causes were verified with vital statistics records. Its most memorable conclusion was that women engaged in prostitution during the last third of the 20th century faced the most dangerous occupational environment in the United States: 50 times more dangerous than that for women who work in liquor stores and 7 times higher than that for *male* taxi cab drivers.[5] The stellar job of analysis and of placing these data in their social and actuarial contexts was the product of Drs. Rothenberg's and Brewer's efforts—which also explains the 3-year delay between data availability and final publication of these exceptional results. Last but not least, our hat is off to Ken Basilio, at the time of the Colorado Springs Vital Statistics Department, whose legendary tenacity in procuring death certificates from rigid and defensive state vital statistics bureaucracies provided the crucial cause of death information.

Prostitution and the sex discrepancy in number of sexual partners

Availability of quality data on prostitute women and their sexual partners in Colorado Springs also permitted testing of Devon Brewer's insight in the late 1990s that prostitution might account for the perplexing and common finding in sexual behaviors surveys that men report substantially more sexual partners than women. This survey discrepancy was consistently noted in countries all over the world and in different stages of development. In short: in heterosexual populations, the numbers of partners reported by men and by women should balance out in the aggregate. This disparity had usually been "explained" by either sex-linked reporting bias (men over-report, and women under-report, partners) or by sample bias (high partner-volume persons not being captured in surveys). Using data from several nationally representative surveys of adults in U.S. households, and data from our contemporaneous survey of Colorado Springs prostitutes and their sexual partners, Brewer was able to show, in a masterful analysis, that prostitution can account for virtually all of the disparity in numbers of partners reported by men and women.[30] He argued that, on the one hand, prostitute women were not likely to be represented in household surveys, since a significant proportion of such women do not live in households but, rather, in venues unlikely to be sampled (jail, prison, motels, rooming houses, homeless shelters, halfway houses). On the other hand, using our data on clients of prostitutes from Project 90 (See Chapter 6), Brewer showed that men were frequently reluctant to acknowledge contact with prostitutes. Adjusting for underrepresentation of prostitute women with large numbers of partners and for clients of prostitutes underreporting such contacts, Brewer mathematically demonstrated that the discrepancy disappears and that the ratio of partners between men and women closely approximates the expected 1:1. This symmetric ratio held for both shorter (one year) and longer (5 years) survey periods. It was the availability and quality of our empiric data that was the critical ingredient for this analysis—an analysis that was reported in one of science's most prestigious journals, *The Proceedings of the National Academy of Sciences.*[30]

Should prostitution be legal?

No discussion of my professional involvement with prostitute women for more than thirty years would be complete without revealing my position during those years on prostitution in society. Queried in 2007 by staff at "Legal Prostitution: Pros and Cons" (*ProCon.org*) I replied:

"As a public health officer I have always maintained neutrality on the legalization issue. I see 3 scenarios: making prostitution illegal (the dominant response almost everywhere); de-criminalizing it (which I view as freedom without responsibility: "I can do my own thing and societal consequences be damned"); and *réglementation* (which gives society control over the rules of engagement and would presumably protect all parties and their interests—including the IRS!). Outlawing prostitution is unrealistic and de-criminalization is irresponsible. Réglementation is realistic, but terribly unlikely to be adopted in America, given the dominant moral climate and professed values. Since legalization is likely to be argued in ideological space and since, therefore, positions will come more from the adrenal than from the cerebral cortex, I view neutrality as the most realistic option."

This sounds like a fence-sitting, cop-out answer. It is. Yet even assuming that legalization were achievable in much of America, I would remain skeptical, if not conflicted. Knowing what I know about what "makes" a prostitute—a mix of "*Les Misérables*" sociology and mental health problems—and what I know of their customers, enough of whom share a similar sociology and also have psychological problems (especially proclivity to violence) I suspect that legalization would not be sufficiently protective of either party, even under controlled circumstances. In my view legalization would attenuate the pathologies associated with prostitution but could never eliminate them. Prostitution would remain a dangerous occupation. And I'm completely open to being proved wrong.

A note on nomenclature: prostitute v. (commercial) sex worker

In an age when "prostitute" has been replaced by the now au courant "sex worker", you may wonder why we have resisted this nomenclature change in our publications. Public health organizations generally view "prostitute" as a disparaging word and that, negative connotations notwithstanding, the word does not properly reflect the "fact" that sex work is a job, not a way of life. (I dispute this "fact" below.) Moreover, in their view, "prostitute" may not fairly describe the involuntary circumstance of women forced into the trade.[31]

We view "prostitute" as a time-honored and scientifically precise term: it simply describes a person who exchanges sex for payment. Negative connotation is not an inherent part of this description. "Sex worker", on the other hand, is imprecise because it can conceal presence of sexual behavior;[31] for example, women who engage in paid telephone sex, or do strip tease, or pose for pornographic venues can be viewed as "sex workers", but is sex part of their work? Most of the time, probably not. Why sacrifice scientific precision for what appears to us to be political correctness?[31] Not to mention that "commercial sex worker" is a (fatuous) tautology.

As for disputing this "fact" I can attest that, during my thirty years on the stroll, I met dozens of prostitutes who took pride in their work and viewed it as a vocation rather than simply a job. Vocations are indeed a way of life. As one of them memorably told me: "different strokes for different folks".

Part 2. Clients of prostitute women: the demand side

No chapter on prostitution would be complete without presenting information on customers of prostitutes: the "johns". In the early years (1970–1985) our primary concern was to rapidly identify and treat STD infected prostitutes; they were important not only because they serviced many men but because, like most infected women, they were not likely to have genital symptoms. Johns were less important because they not only were generally not promiscuous, but because they were likely to experience painful genital symptoms and hence to seek medical attention. In brief: duration of infectiousness for johns was inferred to be much shorter than that for prostitute women.

With the AIDS epidemic came renewed interest in clients of prostitute women. Availability of the HIV antibody test by mid-1985, along with burgeoning interest in the future of the epidemic in heterosexual populations, stimulated a fishing expedition for HIV risk factors; one of many questions asked at the time of blood testing was "Have you had sex with a prostitute since 1978?" Hence, starting in 1985, we were able to collect data on men who admitted to it, whether such exposure occurred in Colorado Springs or elsewhere. Because heterosexual men who did not provide a history of hemophilia or of injecting drug use were rarely positive on the HIV test, we did not single them out for special scrutiny. Such scrutiny only came with our special study of the sexual and street-drug networks of heterosexuals thought to be at high risk for HIV (Project 90: see Chapter 6); this endeavor, implemented during a 5-year period (1988–1992), examined the risks behaviors and HIV status of prostitute women, their street-drug partners, and their paying and non-paying sexual partners. During this period we also sought publicly available data from the Colorado Springs Police Department on arrests for soliciting a prostitute. Hence we had data on clients of prostitutes who had sought HIV testing in our health department clinics or who had been identified by Project 90 (1269 individuals from the two venues) and on arrested johns (923 individuals). (We christened our client computer database "John Thomas" to honor Lady Chatterley's Lover's private parts.) Steve Muth and I had long intended to examine these data with an eye to contribute a "johns" paper to the literature but never got around to it. That turned out to be a blessing in disguise, because Dr. Brewer had thought a lot about johns as he was analyzing the data for the prostitute mortality paper. Specifically, he was curious about the high prostitute women's homicide rate while they were working and,

129

therefore, the likely connection to clients' behavior. Having Dr. Brewer, a rigorous social sciences researcher, get interested in johns and explore features of the demand side of prostitution promised to be methodologically better than what we could do, especially in the absence of financial support for such a study.

Dr. Brewer was able to get support: a grant from the National Institute of Justice. Given adequate external funding, availability of our johns data, and of publicly available information from several police and criminal records databases elsewhere in the United States, he was likely to contribute useful results.

The Devon Brewer Tetralogy:
"johns" under the social science microscope

Our Colorado Springs data had put us in a position to estimate the number of prostitute women in the United States during the 1980s. That estimate represented the supply side of prostitution. It was only natural that an attempt be made to estimate the prevalence of johns, the demand side of prostitution. In a series of brilliantly conceived and analyzed papers,[32–35] Dr. Brewer attempted to 1) derive an estimate of the number of clients of street prostitutes in the United States[32] and of their demographics;[33] 2) determine the extent of prostitution-related homicide, and to describe its perpetrators;[34] and 3) measure the impact, if any, of johns arrests by police.[35] He knew that although we had quality data on the local prostitution scene, our johns data could only

130

play a supporting role in deriving such an estimate. The leading role would have to come from analysis of larger and more diverse sources than we had. Although we provided data and assistance with the interpretation and presentation of these 4 outstanding papers, the lion's share of the methodology and analyses was done by Dr. Brewer and his colleague, Dr. John M. Roberts, Jr.

Estimating the prevalence of male clients of street prostitutes

Previous estimates had principally relied on survey information; Dr. Brewer knew that these were biased, for he had learned from previous analyses[See refs in 32] that men frequently underreported sex with hookers. Hence, he decided to use capture-recapture methods on six available data sets of client arrests that met his specific criteria; these data were available from various large metropolitan areas in the United States. Briefly, his capture-recapture analyses of arrest data indicated that about 2% to 3% of adult males in the United States availed themselves of prostitute women during, say, a 2–5 year interval. Comparing this estimate from the six U. S. metropolitan areas to the estimate he derived from our Colorado Springs data (3.5% of adult males using prostitutes in a given year), he concluded that these were about twice as large as estimates derived from national surveys, which used non-validated self-report information.[32] To satisfy our curiosity, he was specifically able to show that about 5,125 of 146,428 adult men in Colorado Springs had used a prostitute during 1990—a useful and relevant estimate for us indeed, because all epidemiologists need good denominators.

Prostitution-related homicide and its perpetrators

Shocked at the extraordinarily high homicide rate of working prostitutes that he distilled from our prostitute mortality data, Dr. Brewer decided to examine available homicide data to determine the extent, trends, and descriptors of perpetrators, seeing as no prior research on perpetrators of prostitute homicide in the United States had been published. In brief, using nine diverse samples of prostitute homicides—including ours—Dr. Brewer and colleagues[34] were able to estimate that 2.7% of all female homicides in the United States between 1982 and 2000 had occurred in prostitutes. Other major findings were that prostitutes were killed primarily by johns; that johns were killed mainly by prostitutes; and that pimps were killed predominantly by other pimps. The data also indicated that serial killers accounted for at least 35% of all prostitute homicides. (Remarkably, both the extent and perpetrators of prostitute homicide during the 19th century were similar to those observed in the late 20th.) As for the motives of client perpetrators, these included: arguments over the sex/drug transaction, response to the prostitute's attempted robbery of the client, verbal insults from the prostitute, the client's misogyny or hatred of prostitutes, and the client's sadism or other psychopathology. As for homicides committed by prostitutes, these were predominantly associated with robbery or disputes over money, or with characteristics of clients suggestive of vulnerability (attractive target for theft). Pimp homicides committed by other pimps were usually retaliatory "business" killings over turf or with raiding another pimp's prostitute.

Does arrest for soliciting a prostitute act as a deterrent to future soliciting? Yes.

Dr. Brewer was familiar with the literature on criminal offenders, specifically with studies indicating that for many offenders, arrest and penalties do not necessarily decrease a criminal's chances of reoffending. He was naturally interested in assessing a specific deterrent effect: arrest for patronizing a prostitute. Using Colorado Springs data, he intended to see if people arrested by the police for soliciting would be less likely to reoffend than those johns who had been identified through our public health activities but were not known to have been arrested.[35] A lower rate for subsequent arrest would imply that arrest has a deterrent effect on future reoffending and that this could be measured. Analysis of our two sets of johns data (police and public health databases) indicated that arrest reduced the likelihood of reoffending by an impressive 70%. To control for possible displacement (e.g., the johns solicit elsewhere) Brewer examined available data from 4 states; these suggested that only a small proportion (less than 10%) of arrested johns were rearrested in jurisdictions other than the original one.[35]

Reflections

What is notable about our work with prostitutes and their clients in Colorado Springs during the 1970s through 1990s is the phenomenal rate of return on our "investment". Of our many work duties and tasks, I estimate that efforts to contain adverse outcomes of prostitution consumed perhaps five percent of our energies. Yet, as the preceding paragraphs attest, an impressive number of good outcomes resulted from our public health interventions.

Most importantly, the STD burden in prostitute women declined dramatically during these decades. Much of this decline can be attributed to diminished duration of STD infectiousness in infected prostitutes, brought about by relentless efforts to swiftly identify and treat them and their partners; these men, especially their non-paying partners (pimps, boyfriends), were often infected without penile symptoms and served to re-infect the recently treated prostitute unless promptly treated. The combination of vigorous application of the Health Hold Order and of contact tracing to assure treatment of contacts did much to reduce the contribution of prostitution to the overall STD community burden. This I view as our best achievement in the management of the untoward outcomes of prostitution—what we were paid to do by the taxpayer.

The second legacy of our work with prostitutes was accumulation of high quality empiric data which, because published in scholarly journals, may leave a less ephemeral footprint. Our constant presence on the stroll not only helped us to understand their lives, but placed us in a position to ask the right questions. These questions and, above all, our curiosity, frequently stimulated formal investigations to confirm or refute anecdotal impressions. If ever I had entertained a Hollywood or pulp fiction version of prostitution, it was permanently erased by front-line exposure to prostitution in Colorado Springs. Keeping my mouth shut and my eyes and ears open helped me grasp the grim reality and sadness of their often chaotic lives. I retain no illusions about the putative glamour, fun, and adventurism of "The Life". Most people think about prostitution mythologically rather than rationally. In our published work on prostitution you will not find data flavorized by ideological or political considerations. And nowhere is there surrender to fact-corrosive political correctness.

Examining questions of interest to public health and social science researchers using the population, rather than convenience samples, of prostitutes was the special strength of our empiric studies, often made more rigorous by inclusion of non-prostitute comparison women. Most importantly, we were fortunate that both sets of women willingly cooperated, trusting us with the most intimate secrets of their lives. High levels of participation were the norm. It must be said that we encouraged cooperation by clearly articulating how their participation could help public health efforts and the community. We were pleased that they had the nobility to accommodate our requests for information. And we seldom failed to express our gratitude; good manners and courtesy were appreciated.

And did this long-term "investment" ever pay off! Certainly beyond our wildest expectations. Modesty aside, during 3 decades, we contributed some of the best empirical papers on prostitution to the literature. We challenged the received wisdom by showing that what makes a prostitute is likelier to be psychology than sociology. We catalogued the psychological disorders likely to be causal. We presented empiric data to suggest that these psychological problems discouraged prostitutes from availing themselves of rehabilitative services. We presented the first solid estimate of the number of prostitute women in the United States and of their career longevity. We provided the first and only study of mortality in prostitute women using the population, and documenting causes of death with vital statistics records. We used quality empiric data to buttress a plausible solution to a hot button scholarly issue: explaining the discrepancy in reported numbers of sexual partners by heterosexual men and women. Lastly, we provided an evidence-based estimate of the prevalence of clients of prostitute women during the last decades of the 20th century in the United States; a solid analysis of prostitution homicides and its perpetrators; and demonstrated and quantified the deterrent effect on reoffending occasioned by police arrest of prostitute clients.

Altogether, two dozen publications about prostitution appeared in the literature. All in all: a distinctive and distinguished track record.

SIX

MAKING NETS WORK:
THE NETWORK PARADIGM APPLIED TO STD/HIV

"Never underestimate the complexity of social network research"

—Alden Klovdahl

Transplanting the network paradigm

from sociology to epidemiology

Of our many contributions to the STD/HIV field, none has had as much positive impact as our application of the network paradigm to the epidemiology of sexually transmissible diseases.

This interpretive framework was initially imported from sociology by Alden Klovdahl of the Australian National University in 1985[1] as he explored the potential usefulness of network concepts and tools to analyze the original outbreak of HIV in North American homosexual men—the so-called "Patient Zero" outbreak.[2-3] None of us in the Colorado Springs STD/HIV program had heard of this domain of social science theory and research.[4] We were introduced by our colleague Dr. William Darrow, a sociologist working at CDC, who suggested we investigate its usefulness in delineating the risk networks of heterosexuals perceived to be at high risk for HIV infection in our community (prostitute women, injecting drug users, and their sexual and drug partners) and these people's connections to the larger, low-risk heterosexual populations in Middle America. Dr. Darrow had not only graciously accommodated Dr. Klovdahl's request for Patient Zero outbreak data, but had been impressed with his conceptualization and the analysis.[1] My principal interest was in finding solid empirical evidence to test my view that HIV was unlikely to efficiently propagate among heterosexuals who were not injecting street drugs.[5]

For our program, a network approach was a natural fit, which is the reason Dr. Darrow recommended us for this project to his superiors at CDC. Contact tracing and the network approach to studying connections between people were twin disciplines that had emerged in the 1930s, but had been raised apart.[4] Each discipline was apparently unaware of the other's existence. Dr. Darrow knew that the bricks and mortar of network construction in the real world consisted of individuals (nodes) and their relational connections (links). This is precisely what contact tracing was about, and contact tracing had been our epidemiologic modus operandi for nearly two decades—not to mention that we had gotten outstanding results using it. The principal difference was that, in standard contact tracing interviews, the patient being interviewed had been diagnosed with a communicable infection, while in attempting to construct prostitution or injecting drug user networks there was no such stimulus. Would prostitute women and injecting drug users willingly provide personal identifying information about their sexual and drug partners in the absence of communicable disease diagnoses? I was not sure, but because I had a highly experienced and trusted staff, I was willing to try—on one condition: that the study protocols and questionnaires be designed by someone experienced in network methodology. The obvious choice was Dr. Klovdahl. He gladly accepted the challenge. And this is how the influential Project 90 was born. ("Project 90" identified blood test specimens collected from our participants to laboratory staff who processed them at the CDC in Atlanta.)

A. Our Million-Dollar study:

network architecture as transmission destiny

Project 90 was the first prospective study of the influence of network structure on infectious disease transmission. The basic proposition being empirically tested was that the configuration of connections between people would have consequences for either facilitating or constraining STD/HIV transmission, above and beyond people's risk behaviors for transmission. In brief: the social organization of relationships ("network"), specifically risky relationships ("risk network"), was predicted to significantly influence patterns of infectious disease propagation.[1] Were this true—that network architecture facilitated or constrained transmission pathways—then knowledge of this topography could be used to intervene in community STD/HIV transmission.

Networks are typically depicted as nodes (individuals) connected by links (risk relationships) in 2- or 3-dimensional visualizations ("sociograms"[6]), which can provide powerful visual cues about the natural world of STD/HIV transmission. As well, concepts and methods from mathematical graph theory are commonly used to analyze network properties and data.[7–8]

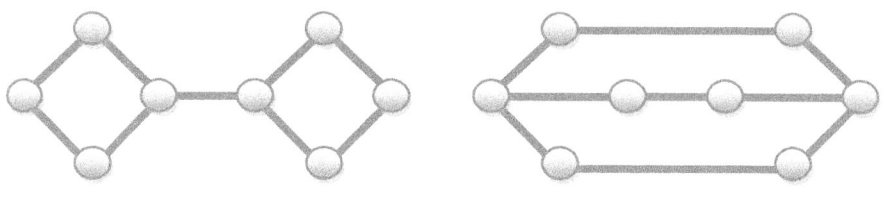

Network A   Network B

Figure 4: Influence of network conformation on diffusion of infections associated with sexual or injecting drug-use behaviors

Each network has exactly the same number of persons (nodes), the same number of risky behaviors (links), the same numbers of partners (2 persons in each network have 3 partners each, while the rest each have 2)—and yet diffusion of infection is facilitated in Network B (in two steps from the index person on the left, 7 persons are exposed) compared to network A, where only half are exposed in 2 steps from the index person on the left.

Additionally, to prevent half the population from being exposed, only one link needs to be severed in Network A (the middle horizontal), compared to 3 in Network B (all horizontal links).

Illustration by Alden S. Klovdahl, as it appeared in our article in *Bulletin de Méthodologie Sociologique*.[8] Graphic layout by Steve Muth, Oct 2015.

Though he lived and worked in Australia, Dr. Klovdahl initially made several short visits, starting in the autumn of 1987, to Colorado Springs and later spent six months in residence to develop the tools for the proposed network investigation locally. Colorado Springs was selected not only because of its expertise in contact tracing and its successful association with elusive and disenfranchised populations, but also because HIV reporting was mandatory in Colorado and HIV cases were actively monitored in a relatively small and well bounded geographic space. In the absence of mandatory HIV reporting, any network study of HIV transmission would be missing blood on the transmission tracks, as it were.

Recruiting high-risk heterosexual populations in Colorado Springs

Because of their high-volume, high risk sexual practices (e.g., anal intercourse) and frequent injection of street-drugs, prostitutes were deemed high risk heterosexuals, along with their sexual and street-drug partners. The second group of heterosexuals deemed at elevated risk were street-drug injectors, along with their sexual and street-drug partners.

Dr. Klovdahl, who was familiar with network sampling methods, considered alternative study designs and persuaded us that the most viable approach, given our local situation, was to aim for the entire target populations as a starting point. Enrolling a convenience sample of prostitutes was not necessary because, given their relatively small number, and an even smaller number of non-paying partners (pimps, boyfriends), aiming to enroll these entire populations was a reasonable expectation. In brief, we were facing manageable numbers: 217

prostitute women were eventually observed during the 40-month enrollment period, and roughly half had pimps or boyfriends.

At the start, however, the immediate obstacles were not knowing how many injecting drug users and johns (men who patronized prostitutes) lived in our community, because local estimates were not available. Dr. Klovdahl suggested using site-based recruiting, augmented by link-tracing. What this meant is that we would recruit in-treatment injecting drug users at the health department methadone maintenance clinic (site recruiting), of which there were 65 in late 1987, and ask them to nominate fellow injectors, in- or out-of treatment, whom we could then attempt to enroll (link-tracing). Johns could be recruited in the local prostitution soliciting areas (site recruiting) and through clients identified by prostitutes (including link-tracing, especially of "regulars", because they were potentially easier to locate, unlike casual clients). Lastly, people who were named as contacts by more than one participant were eligible for recruitment; they were called "cross-links" because it was thought that such potential participants would increase the probability of tying network regions together.[9]

Ethical and legal considerations

Crucially, our Institutional Review Boards and Ethics Committees allowed us the freedom to make our own selections from lists of names provided by participants for subsequent "link-tracing" interviews. This imposed special responsibilities on us, reflected in the design of the interview and in the selections we eventually made; a principal concern was not exposing participants or their named partners to possible breaches of confidentiality. In a conventional sampling design, persons to be interviewed next in a network study are made by participants in the study, not by the researchers. By having the freedom to choose, for example, multiply-connected people (those named by several different participants), we could increase the likelihood of seeing connected regions within the entire Colorado Springs networks. Moreover, because this was a pioneering study in the STD/HIV domain, we felt it was important to delineate and discuss the ethical and legal issues involved in network research.[9–10]

Project 90 data collection instruments

Klovdahl did not intend to simply describe static networks—a mere cross section of reality. He felt it was crucial to study networks as they changed through time. What especially interested him was being able to observe the evolution of, say, purely social-to-risky relationships, and vice-versa. To assess the impact of changes in network configuration over time, participants were to be offered interviews every year for up to 5 years to discern dynamic patterns of living arrangements, health problems, and risk behaviors. Starting in the third year of the study, enrollees were offered remuneration: $15 for the initial, $25 for the second, and $35 for any subsequent, interview. None was offered during the first 2 years because we did not deem it necessary, and because we thought it might bias enrollment; as we later learned, it didn't.[10-11] The money was, however, an attractive incentive for participants to return for subsequent annual interviews.

Because both behavioral and network data were required to describe nodes and links, participants were asked to respond to two survey instruments. The behavioral questionnaire consisted of about 140 items, including demographic data, pertinent medical history, knowledge about HIV, street-drug use, and sexual history. While the main period of interest was the preceding year, several items (sex and drugs) covered the previous five years. It took approximately a half-hour to complete this face-to-face questionnaire, which was designed by more than a dozen experienced researchers.[12] No tape recording or video equipment was used.

The network questionnaire required about an hour to complete; details are available elsewhere.[8-9,11,13] It consisted of recording the names of the participant's social, sexual, and street drug (especially drug-injecting) partners for the prior six months. Detailed questions were asked about each nominated partner: sex, age, ethnicity, occupation, full name/nicknames, address, phone numbers, nature and strength of relationship (on a scale of 1 to 10), sexual exposures, and drug practices—and to record each named partner's sex and drug behavior, if known, with the other named partners. Identifying the participant's social partners helped delineate their social network, while sex and drug questions delineated their HIV risk network. Participants were then asked to provide a blood specimen (30 ml) to be tested at the CDC for

HIV, hepatitis-B, syphilis, and human T-lymphotropic virus (HTLV). Both questionnaires and blood testing were repeated at each subsequent annual interview. Lastly, participants who were partners of prostitutes were asked an additional fifteen questions about their sexual practices with these women and about their motivation for soliciting them.

Succeeding beyond expectation:
Project 90 results and impact on the field

The critical initial finding was that members of the populations of interest—those engaging in illegal behaviors—prostitute women, street-drug users, and johns—were willing to provide, for research purposes, detailed identifying information on their social, drug, and sexual partners. Although in retrospect this may seem obvious, in any network study there is always the question as to whether prospective participants are willing and able to cooperate, even if pilot trials had been done. In our Colorado Springs study, our target participants willingly revealed the most intimate secrets of their, and their partners', lives.[9] Absent this cooperation, Project 90 would have collapsed at the starting gate. One can never be sufficiently appreciative for this kind cooperation and participant nobility.

Participant recruitment

Baseline recruitment of participants began in May 1988 and ended 40 months later, in August 1991. Of the 1079 people assessed as eligible for enrollment during this interval, 595 (55%) were successfully enrolled. The principal difficulty consisted of locating these members of largely elusive or hidden populations. Their fluid lifestyle and impermanent domiciles also made it challenging to locate participants for annual re-interviews. Seventy-two percent of those meeting the study criteria who were not enrolled (348 of 494) were either not located, or were not asked to participate because so doing might have tipped them off about how we got their name and, therefore, compromised our participant-informant's confidentiality. For example, if a "john" was known to frequent only one prostitute, seeking to interview him could have led, correctly or not, to his inferring that it was his preferred prostitute who revealed his name to us. Knowledge of this (and similar) possibility was a particularly heavy responsibility we shouldered for the duration of the study.[10] Fewer than twenty percent of eligible people approached (136 of 731) actually declined to participate. The 133 participating prostitutes represented three-fifths of the 217 recorded during the enrollment period, while the 766 street-drug injectors identified as a consequence of being named in interviews represented half of the rough contemporary estimate of street-drug injectors in Colorado Springs.[9]

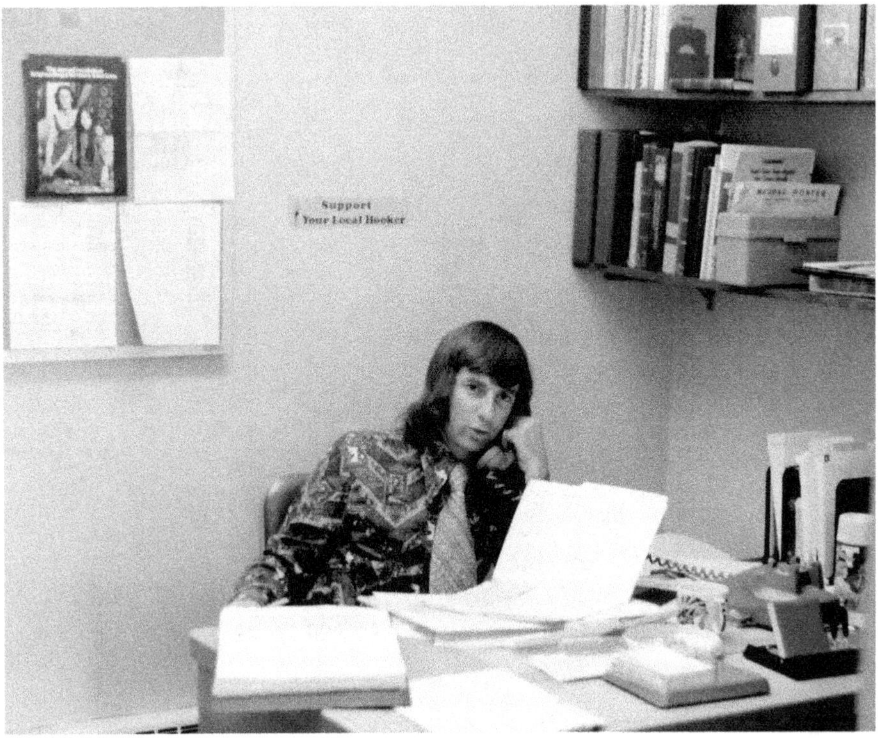

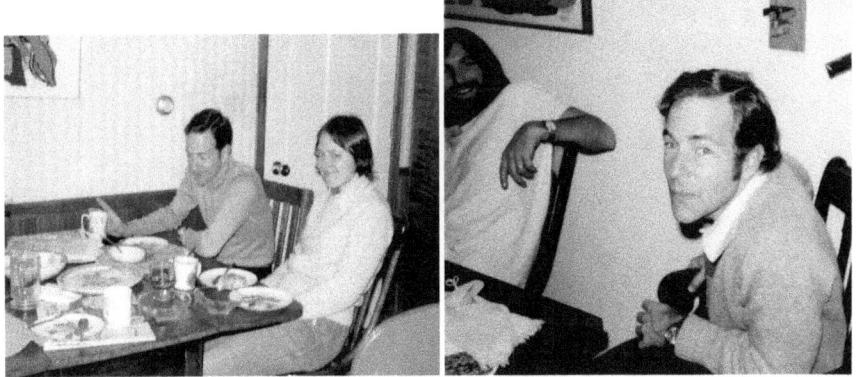

The author reviewing clinic charts in the (small and sole) VD Program office, circa 1974. Note bumper sticker on back wall.

The brilliant and athletic Dr. Richard Rothenberg next to his audiophile (and first) wife Carol in John's kitchen, 1979. Rich and John plot their next move (right).

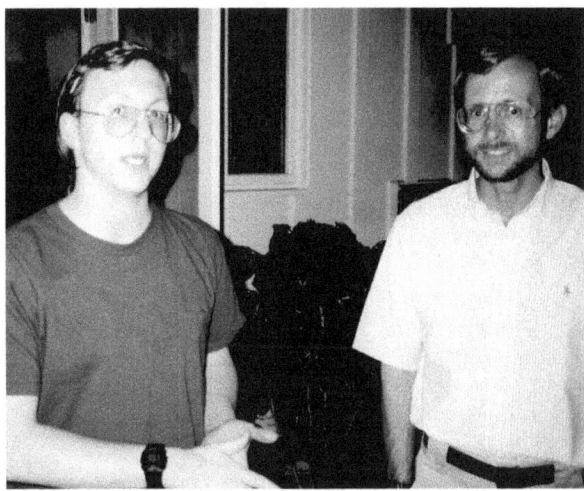

Masterful Information Technology guru Stephen Q. Muth (left) and wise-scholarly manager of Project 90, Donald E. Woodhouse, JD on my patio, 1993.

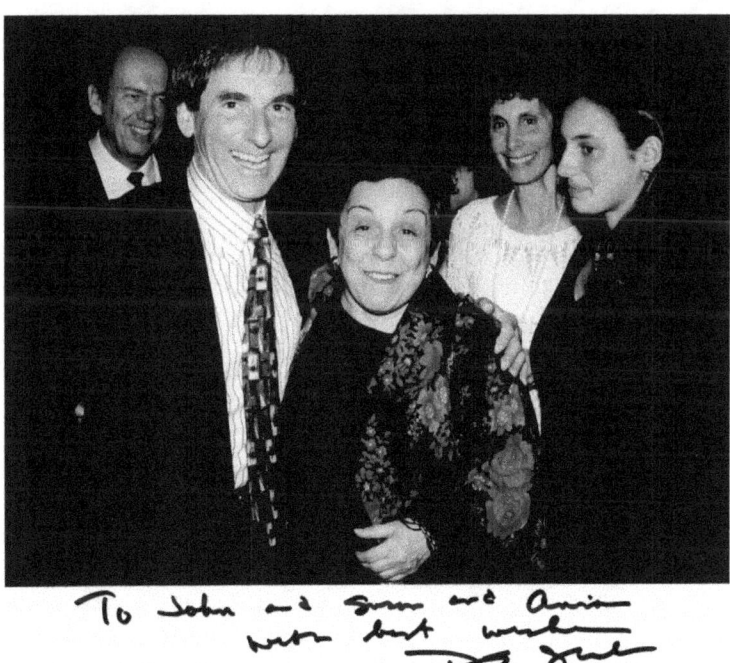

Secretary of Health and Human Services Donna Shalala attending the American Medical Association's 1993 Nathan Davis Awards banquet in Washington D.C., congratulating the author as an award recipient, flanked by his wife Susan and daughter Anna, early 1994. Dr. John Muth is behind, on the left.

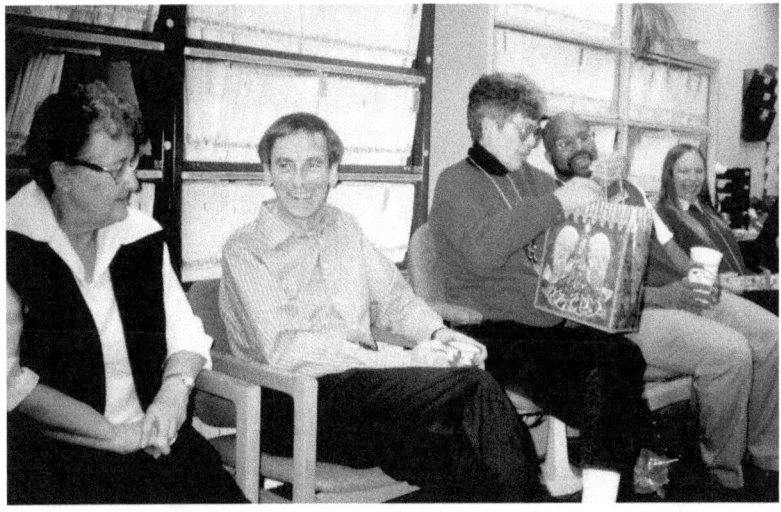

Holiday Season party in chart room of STD Clinic, December 1998. From left: The redoubtable and indefatigable Helen P. Zimmerman, me, data entry clerk Patricia Cox, and contact tracers Dave Green and Lynanne Plummer-Phillips.

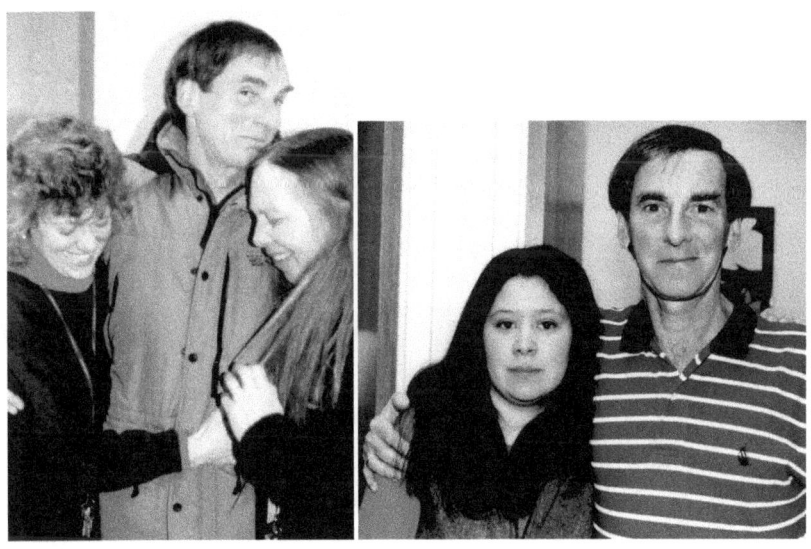

The author, flanked by program supervisors Helen L. Zimmerman-Rogers (STD) and Lynanne Plummer-Phillips (HIV & Blood-borne infections), on the eve of his departure in January 2001. The proud author at right, with soon-to-be HIV & Blood-borne infections supervisor Tammy Maldonado, the brains behind the (manual, paper-based) identity-matching effort in Project 90.

.

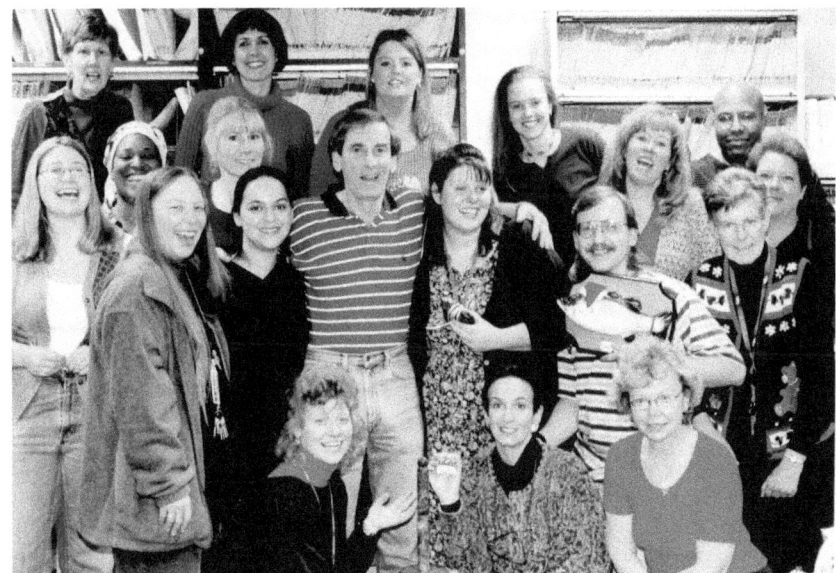

Virtually the entire STD/HIV Programs staff the month of my retirement, January 2001. Front row (left to right): Lynanne Plummer-Phillips, Pamela Montoya, Helen Zimmerman-Rogers, Judith Reynolds, MD (holding condoms), Trudi Tong. Second (and wavy) row, left to right: Shana Hurlbutt-Sanderson, Andrea Dubose, Patricia Malone, me, Julie Higgins, Steve Muth (holding Santa fish), Patricia Cox. Back row (left to right): Linda Coughlin, Taunia Ryan, Dayna Dorobiala, Heather Stites, Cheryl Justis, Dave Green, and Lani Fair.

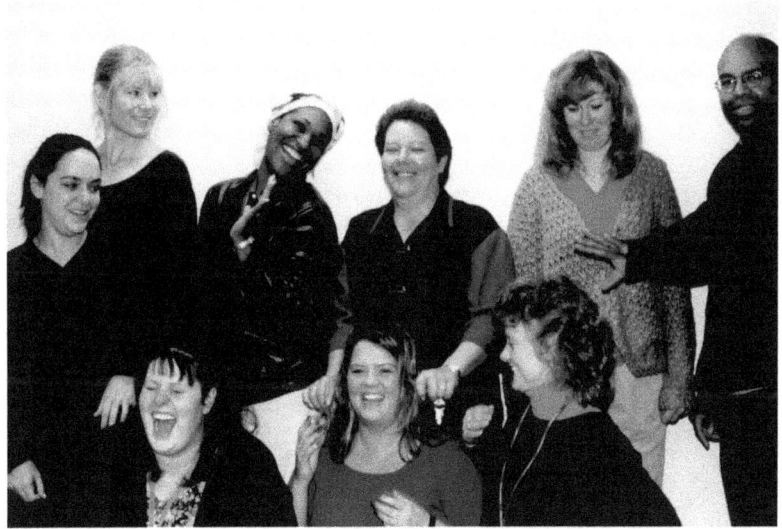

My enthusiastic and joyful STD/HIV staff (because of my imminent departure?) January 2001.

Total number of unique nodes, risky links,
HIV positives, and components identified

Overall, in 1091 interviews (595 baseline, 288 second, 135 third, and 73 fourth/fifth, interviews), 8759 unique individuals were identified, connected by 31,147 links. Network analysis revealed how closely-linked the populations of interest were: four-fifths (7151 of the 8759 people) comprised one single giant connected component.[9,14] In graph-theoretic terms, a connected component is a region of a network in which everyone is connected, directly or indirectly, to everyone else by a path (sequence of links) of some length. This finding was powerful evidence to undermine the assumption frequently used in epidemic mathematical models that social, drug, or sexual associations are random mixing events; at-risk populations are definitely not amorphous entities where people randomly interact. Beyond this giant connected component, there were also 116 smaller components, no member of which had any demonstrable social, sexual, or drug-using link to any member of the largest component. Of the total 31,147 links, about one-fifth were classified as risky relationships for HIV transmission.

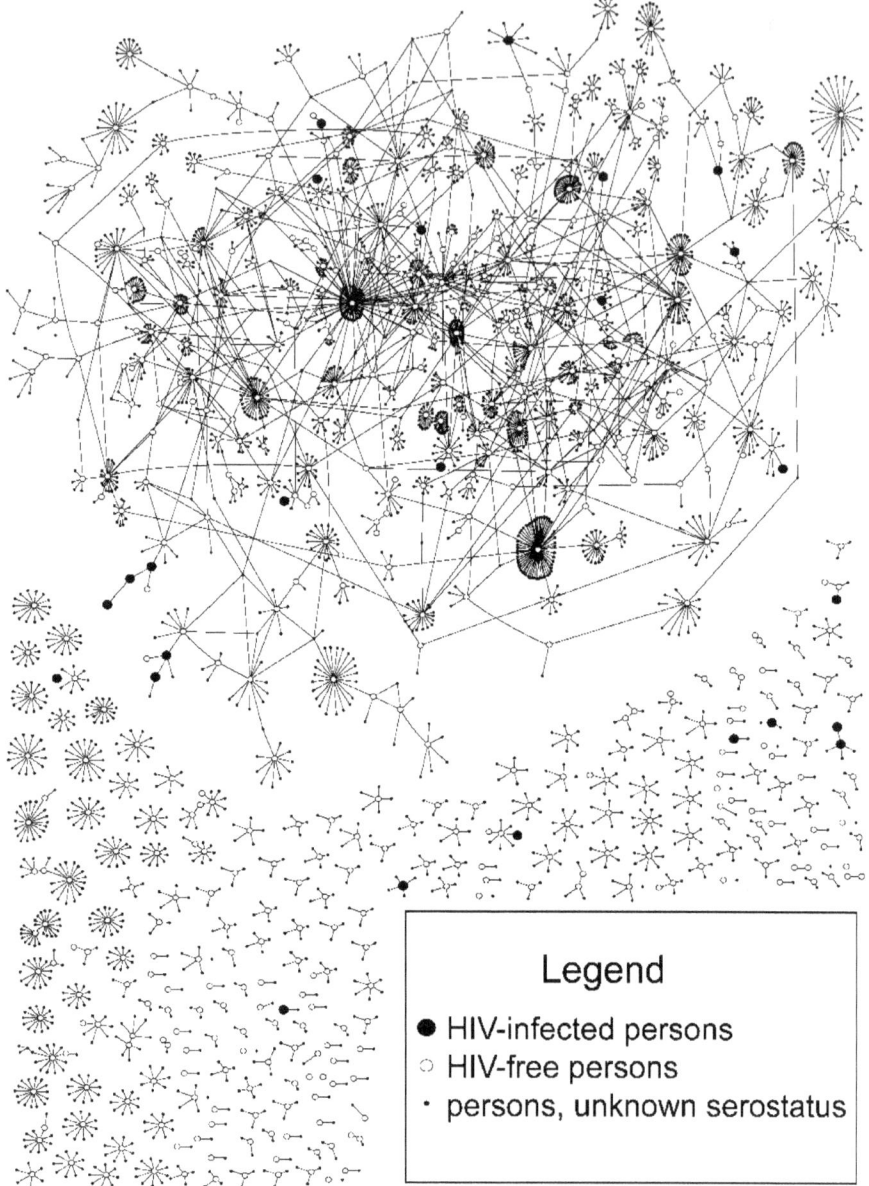

Figure 5: Recent-risk network (sex/needle connections) showing location of HIV-infected persons in Project 90, 1988–93

Reprinted from our Oxford University Press chapter illustration.[9] Original graphic by Steve Muth.

By design, only participants and named partners who were, or became, participants were blood tested. In all, 36 people were shown to be HIV-positive, either by direct testing or by matching names to our Program's HIV-positives database. Only 4 were assessed as having acquired HIV during the study period;[9,14] 3 provided histories of injecting drug use—2 men and a street prostitute—and the fourth, also a woman, provided a history of anal intercourse with an injecting drug user. As for their location within networks, not only did the giant component contain fewer than half of the identified HIV-positive persons, but those who were HIV-positive tended to occupy peripheral, rather than central, positions (i.e., they received low network centrality scores). For example, more than half of HIV-positive persons were located, in network terms, in much smaller components, ranging in size from 2 to 24 people, components not connected to each other or to the giant component. HIV infection failed to reach the giant network's most central core, where pathways that would have allowed transmission were much more numerous than in its peripheral regions. The association between the peripheral locations of HIV-infected people in network regions characterized by risky relationships, and the dearth of observed HIV transmission during the study interval in Colorado Springs was the first prospective demonstration of the influence of network structure on infectious disease propagation.[15] As I concluded: "Just as language can be conceptualized as a flow of words structured by rules of grammar, so may epidemics be viewed as a flow of microbes structured by the 'grammar' of social network structures".[15]

Yet this is not to discount or ignore the potential role of human intercession, for in this study we were unable to ascertain the extent, if any, to which HIV-positive persons voluntarily isolated themselves from, or were marginalized by, others.

Dynaflow:[16] Changing architecture of networks over time

Project 90's prospective design provided the opportunity to describe network change and study its impact. The changing configuration of risk networks over time was thought to be important for a clearer understanding of STD/HIV transmission dynamics. In brief, analysis of network changes over time in Colorado Springs confirmed the conclusion derived from analysis of the cross-sectional (static as opposed to dynamic) picture of our networks: network structure influences infectious disease propagation over and above effects of individual risk behaviors.[1] In different words, risk behavior is what a person does and risk configuration is the influential structural context in which it is practiced.[17–18]

This pioneering and masterful analysis was principally done by Dr. Rothenberg.[19] Using data from participants who were interviewed at multiple (two or three) time points, he showed that both risk behaviors and risk configurations in Colorado Springs changed in the direction of decreasing risk. Overall, dynamic changes resulted in both an increase in the number of components and in a decrease in their size—which, simply, means that network density and connectivity diminished over time, presenting fewer opportunities for sustaining STD/HIV transmission. Membership in networks varied considerably over time, a not unexpected result in view of the activity and nature of relationships within these groups. Overall, sexual connections were more stable than other types of relationships, and street-drug using partners were the least stable. Generally, persons in large network regions experienced greater partner turnover than those in small networks. Importantly, injecting drug users reported fewer sharing partners over time and, indeed, many reported that they no longer shared needles. This reduction in needle-sharing was accompanied by significant network structural changes, in the direction of less connectivity and lower network density.

Given the available Project 90 data, we were regrettably unable to measure the extent to which noted changes might have been due to our public health interventions (stimulating risk behavior modifications) or to an inherent tendency of networks to undergo spontaneous changes. Be that as it may, this analysis was the first empirical demonstration of dynamic network structural changes being associated with observed infectious disease (in this particular instance, lack of) propagation. Notably, these results were important in stimulating social scientists to re-examine purely behavioral explanations for STD/HIV transmission: risk behavior is a necessary but not sufficient condition for STD/HIV propagation at the population level.[17–19]

Network centrality measures as
surrogates for STD/HIV transmission potential

To further examine the influence of network structure on infectious disease propagation, Dr. Rothenberg used centrality measures commonly employed in social network analysis. Originally intended by sociologists to measure social position, influence, and support in human relations, Dr. Rothenberg's intellectual transplant represents the first testing of network centrality measures in epidemiology.[20] He was specifically interested in examining the relationship between network prominence and STD/HIV transmission potential, meaning: were the people occupying central positions in a network better situated to be successful transmitters than those in non-central positions? Using Project 90 data from the single largest, giant connected component (where there was a path of some length from every person to every other person), he tested eight different measures of network centrality against data on participants whose risk behaviors and practices (e.g., street-drug use, sexual practices, injecting drug use) ranged from high- to lower-risk. He found that although each of the eight measures differed in their theoretical underpinnings and in computational methods, they produced similar results, correctly classifying people with high-risk transmission behavioral profiles and, more importantly, confirming that HIV-infected people in Colorado Springs' high-risk heterosexual populations occupied network positions of low centrality. Hence network centrality measures provided further support for the crucial role played by structural elements in infectious disease propagation. It follows that some measures of centrality could be useful surrogates for disease transmission potential; this in itself has implications for the design and implementation of more focused, rather than more scattered, interventions.

Plotting an actual network in real geographic space

Of the many contributions spawned by analysis of Project 90 data, one is especially exciting: visualizing network connections in geographical (as opposed to graph) space. This tour de force was principally achieved by Steve Muth and Dr. Rothenberg—dueling intellectual banjos.

Although both Dr. Rothenberg and I had demonstrated 2 decades prior [21–22] (see Chapter Two) that gonorrhea was a neighborhood disease by showing the compact geographical and social distribution of such cases, and had inferred that such tight clustering reflected homophily (similar people tend to live in similar neighborhoods and to select partners from within their neighborhoods), the geographic data on participant-partner pairs (dyads) had not been available to conclusively support this view. In simplest social network terms, a dyad consists of 2 persons who are connected by one relationship, such as a married couple. The aim of their analysis, using Project 90 data, was to examine the relationship between social (how closely people are connected by both risk behaviors and emotional attachment) and geographic (how closely people are connected by actual distance as the crow flies) distance. Again, they used data from the largest Project 90 connected component, which was shown to contain nearly 4,000 dyadic relationships.[23] To measure social distance, they calculated the shortest number of network steps—degrees of separation, if you will—between any pair of people in the connected component. Strength of relationship was derived from participants' rating, on a scale of 1 to 10, of how close they felt to each person they nominated. For geographic distance, they measured the "as the crow flies" distance between each participant-partner pair (dyad).

The remarkable result was how compact these distances were, echoing a report from Baltimore a few years earlier using gonorrhea contact tracing data [24] —although theirs was not a complete network. In Colorado Springs, the average geographic distance between each member of the 4,000 dyads was about 3.3 miles; considering that the average distance between any two people in Colorado Springs has been measured as about 9 miles, one can infer that high-risk heterosexuals in Project 90 were, on average, 2.7 times closer to each other than were members of the general population. Specifically, slightly more than half of the dyads were geographically separated by 2.5 or fewer miles. The shortest average distance was among dyads that shared a sexual relationship and street-drug needles (2 miles); dyads sharing sex only were separated by almost twice that distance (3.7 miles); dyads involving a prostitute and a paying partner were separated by a similar interval (3.8 miles); and dyads sharing needles only, by 2.5 miles. Thus, all geographic distances among high-risk dyads were considerably smaller than the average of 9 miles for the undifferentiated general population. As for social distance, about half of dyads were separated by only 3 to 6 network steps (Range: 1 to 14) and were separated by an average geographic distance of only 1.25 to 5 miles. Both social and geographic distances were strongly correlated and compact. This turns out to be good news for the application of public health interventions aiming to reduce street-drug abuse and unsafe sex in populations at high risk for adverse health outcomes: tailored, focused interventions within highly bounded socio-geographical spaces are likely to be more effective and cheaper than diffuse efforts in the general population. Given this evidence, the problem of reaching those at elevated risk suddenly was deemed much more manageable than before. Finally, the very special feature of this analysis was the mapping of an entire risk network in geographic space.[23]

Using geography to gauge ascertainment bias: assessing sample representativeness

As with the geographical analysis of network data just outlined, the investigation described below was also made possible by availability of precise coordinates in real geographic space, based on Global Positioning System (GPS) technology. A nagging methodological question was the extent to which our Project 90 findings might have been biased because we were unable to recruit more participants from the pool of eligible people. Recall that only 595 (55%) of the 1079 people who met our eligibility criteria were enrolled and interviewed.

Traditionally, comparability of participants with non-participants was assessed by contrasting standard demographic characteristics, such as age, sex, ethnicity, occupational category, income level, and educational attainment; such comparisons may not be sufficient to indicate whether or not participants of a specific subgroup are similar to non-participants in the same subgroup. Because people who are alike tend to live in neighborhoods with people who share similar characteristics ("Nearby things tend to be alike" is Tobler's First Law of Geography [25]), using geographic information to visualize the distributions of participants and non-participants in real space might provide insight about network sample representativeness not reflected by demographic data alone. I thus asked Steve Muth to explore how this could be done.

Muth eventually devised a technique to compute average GPS distances from a central point in geographic space, using both participant and non-participant land addresses for members of each subgroup of interest, and displaying them visually using a rotational moving box plot[26] statistical device. Although the demographic data distributions, especially those for men, tended to differ between participants and non-participants, the geographical coordinates distributions were similar for both participants and non-participants (both distributions varied considerably from that of the general population in being much more compact and focal). Participants and non-participants were concentrated in the central parts of Colorado Springs; superimposed, both groups shared a 70% geographic overlap.

We now knew that our participants tended to be drawn from the same areas of town as non-participants; in other words, because "nearby things tend to be alike", there was a stronger argument now that participants could now be viewed as representative of the underlying populations of interest: high-risk heterosexuals in Colorado Springs. Thus Project 90 data analysis made yet another contribution to network science by providing an additional tool for investigating network sampling representativeness.

Contrasting network configuration
with observed STD/HIV transmission

Project 90's aim was to obtain empirical evidence that network structure strongly influenced infectious disease propagation by facilitating or constraining transmission pathways. Moreover, we believed that knowledge of such network topography could be used to develop more effective interventions designed to prevent STD/HIV transmission in our community. Managed by Donald Woodhouse, Project 90 convincingly associated constrained network conformation with lack of HIV transmission. Yet, ours was only a sample of one—one city, one large network. The argument would be much more convincing if one could also associate actual disease transmission with facilitating or constraining network structure. The opportunity to compare and contrast constraining versus facilitating network features in context of STD transmission presented itself a few years later.

In 1996, a group of adolescents near a large Southern U.S. city were involved in intense sexual activity during several months that resulted in successful transmission of ten syphilis cases in their milieux.[27] Network analysis of the contact tracing data indicated increasing network cohesion over time; for example, the number of components decreased from about a dozen small ones to a single large connected component comprising 95 people (along with a single component containing only 4 people). Importantly, during the outbreak, a strong relationship was noted between the increasing complexity of both large and small network structures and the timing of syphilis diagnoses. Sexual behaviors did not change appreciably after outbreak containment, but its social organization did; there was a marked reduction in group sex, which had provided a transmission turbo effect, as it were. Recall that the opposite process was observed in Project 90. One large connected component fragmented over time into a number of smaller ones, resulting in an increasingly (structurally) anemic transmission environment; only one HIV transmission among recruited index participants was observed during the entire 5-year study period. These findings clearly supported the (at the time, minority of) researchers who were calling for reevaluation of purely behavioral explanations of STD/HIV transmission. Importantly, there was increasing recognition of the need to develop and test network-based and network-informed interventions. For example, it was argued that segmentation of risk networks and, consequently, reduction in likely transmission, could be achieved by closing (or making them safer) gay bathhouses where men meet to have multiple sexual relationships, and by closing shooting galleries (or making them safer) where street-drug injectors share drugs and injecting paraphernalia. Another network structural intervention would be to encourage substitution of sexual concurrency (overlapping partners) with serial monogamy, for the network conformation of the latter would be much less permissive of transmission than the former.[28]

Necessity as mother of invention

Project 90 was implemented in the early days of network analysis software development. Most available programs could not accommodate large numbers of nodes or/and perform complex network calculations, such as solving high-order powers of a matrix, or inverting matrices. Initially we were able to use a Fortran program written by David Carrick and Ros Omodei, modified by Klovdahl (called Macronet [29]) to calculate some basic properties of large networks. But additional calculations were essential to establish nodal prominence (the centrality and degree of connectivity of any individual in the network). Steve Muth recruited his brilliant mathematician friend Kurt Foster to help tackle this problem. Their solution was to reduce computational intensity, if possible. As it turned out, three types of centrality measures (viz., Katz, Hoede, and Hubbel) contained computational shortcuts, which involved a return to the original matrix formulation featured at the beginning of their papers.[30] Software developers had, up to this point, overlooked the fact that these scores could be computed by adding the first few terms of a polynomial instead of computing a matrix inverse—a calculation that is still impractical on today's PCs as network size approaches 10,000 nodes. This achieved the desired result—estimating the relative importance of individuals in our large networks—in far less time, using available computer crunching power and data storage space. This shortcut has been incorporated into the current network analysis software NEGOPY. Additional SAS macro programming routines were adapted from techniques developed by Dr. Rothenberg to automate more esoteric network analyses.

Project 90 difficulties and costs

Project 90 presented many difficult operational and administrative obstacles; these are detailed elsewhere.[9,31] Chief among them was the dearth of network analysis software tools powerful enough to accommodate large numbers of nodes; of adequate network visualization tools; and of personal computers powerful enough to perform complex network calculations, especially matrix inversions. To make up for these serious deficits, our inventive information systems manager, Steve Muth, devised ingenious algorithms using the SAS software package and adapted useful features of the few available—and, at the time, underdeveloped—network graphics software programs (see Appendix 1). Visualizing networks in 3-dimensional space was essential for HIV transmission-potential pattern recognition.

Lack of adequate network analysis software notwithstanding, the Colorado Springs staff seriously underestimated both the complexity of analyzing social network data and the stamina of our sponsoring agency, the CDC.[9] With the retirement from CDC of Project 90 officer Dr. Darrow in mid-1991, CDC's interest in our network endeavor waned and they pressured us to discontinue enrolling new participants; to concentrate on completing follow-up interviews; and to prepare manuscripts for publication. CDC did not have the foggiest notion of how time consuming data clean-up and collation would be, nor did we have the in-house expertise to analyze complex network data. Fortunately, in the early 1990s, the National Institute on Drug Abuse (NIDA) was expressing interest in the network paradigm. It was my good fortune to share a cab to the airport in Yokohama, Japan in August 1994—site of the International AIDS Conference—with Dr. Richard Needle who, upon hearing my story, encouraged me to apply for funding from his agency to discipline the data and support data analysis. Dr. Needle was with the Division of Epidemiology and Prevention Research at NIDA. For five years of Project 90 data collection, CDC paid $786,442, while the two-year NIDA grant paid $366,456; thus Project 90's total cost to the taxpayer was $1,152,898—a productive Million-Dollar study indeed.

B. Application of network analysis to our other STD/HIV datasets

Analyzing Project 90 turned out to be a dress rehearsal for applying network analytic tools to data we were routinely collecting in our daily work doing STD/HIV contact tracing. Such data, consisting of infected people (nodes) naming other people exposed by sexual contact (links), lent themselves quite naturally to network analysis. As detailed in previous chapters, network analysis identified the 107 principal transmitters in the 1991 gonorrhea outbreak in crack cocaine gangs;[32] the 39 people—four-fifths of whom were HIV-positive gay men, including five who were also injecting drug users—who, in the early 1980s, formed "ground zero" for HIV propagation in Colorado Springs;[33] and the 40% (1736 of 4359) of young people who resided in local chlamydia core transmission networks.[34] Yet our principal interest was in continuing to empirically explore the association between sexual network conformation and epidemic phase[34–35] (is incidence stable, waxing, or waning?) using STD/HIV contact tracing data. Along these lines, we were able to reveal the geometry of rapid transmission—"cyclic" connections associated with intense STD transmission in the crack cocaine gangs' milieu;[32–33] the increasingly fragmented components structure of HIV sexual networks during the last 15 years of the 20th century in Colorado Springs and its association with rapidly declining HIV incidence;[33,35] and the linear branching geometry (devoid of cyclic connections), and severely fragmented components distribution, of chlamydia sexual networks and their association with stable-to-declining incidence in Colorado Springs.[34,36] These findings provided additional evidence for the primal role played by network configuration (how people connect in sexual space) and confirmed that sexual behaviors alone do not, ipso facto, correspond with actual risk of infection or transmission.

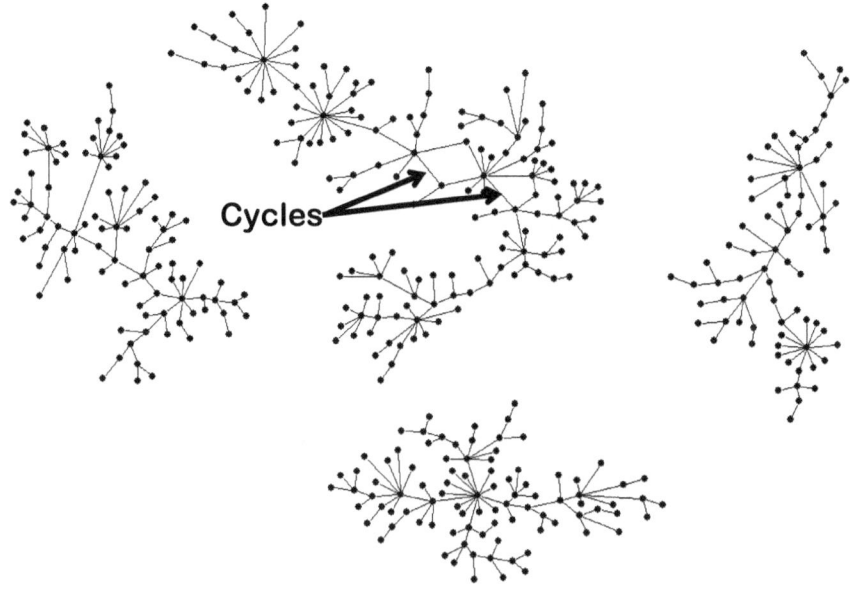

Figure 6: Graph of the 4 largest networks of chlamydia-exposed persons in Colorado Springs, 1996-1999

Original illustration by Steve Muth October 2015, and is based on our article in *Sexually Transmitted Infections*.[34]

C. Other voices: Project 90 data analyses by exogenous researchers

The availability of a large and non-static network data set presented academic researchers with the opportunity to test their theories using real world data. There were few similarly complete datasets anywhere, because such data were notoriously difficult and labor-intensive to collect. Hence we recognized a special responsibility to provide access to these data for scholars. We constructed Project 90 data sets, de-identified (sanitized of personal identifiers), with codebooks and made them freely available as soon as they had been cleaned of errors of commission and omission. This task took about two years to complete after termination of field data collection in 1992. Enhanced sets took a few years longer, for we had to solve the problems of segmenting data into longitudinal cohorts and various sampling categories (for statistical estimation). Also we had to obtain precise geographical coordinates. (GIS geocoding of local addresses by our city-county governments was not available until May of 1997.) It is worth mentioning that the principal sampling question of interest—what is the minimum amount of network information needed to rapidly and reliably assess network structure—was so complex that it has thus far resisted the efforts of many adroit statisticians to solve. Were economical, user-friendly network sampling techniques available, more investigators would undertake network studies instead of being deterred by the daunting task of full network ascertainment.

We also had selfish motives for offering free access: outside researchers would be asking different questions than we—not to mention that we did not have sufficient expertise in specialized domains of inquiry, particularly mathematical modeling and statistical estimation. Last but not least, we felt a profound obligation to honor our participants' cooperation; failing to have the data thoroughly analyzed, whether by us or by those with different expertise, would have been to seriously undervalue participant goodwill, trust, and openness.

As of this writing (2015), nearly twenty scholarly analyses have used Project 90 data to test specific theories, many of which address issues in statistical sampling of networks.[37–53] Because participants in network research are not usually randomly selected, the standard statistical assumptions used to make inferences from random samples of individuals in situations with known underlying distributions are often not appropriate.[37–43] Other studies focused on assessing the reliability and validity of participant responses,[44–45] and on the robustness of traditional tools used in network analysis.[46–47] Results were published in respected scholarly journals.[37–53]

The sincerest form of flattery

Project 90 was a path-breaking investigation of the impact of network conformation on the transmission of infectious disease agents. Remarkably, it was successfully implemented not by trained researchers, but by lower-level government functionaries—local STD/HIV shoe-leather contact tracers with no prior experience in the management of network studies. This was a strength, for had I been cognizant of the daunting complexities such studies entailed, it is unlikely that I would have accepted the challenge. Ignorance was bliss. Especially helpful was our health department's administrative culture under the exceptionally gifted director, Dr. John Muth, who encouraged ideas and data-based innovation during his tenure from 1980 to 1997 in the independent Colorado Springs health department. And it has certainly not been lost on me that, as the county's health officer, he could have denied approval for implementing Project 90. One can accomplish much in a supportive work environment that is neither hierarchically nor bureaucratically rigid. Dr. Muth was patient, never pressing for quick results, a style unlike that seen in often politically-pressured public health bureaucracies.

Other researchers soon followed in our footsteps, principally Drs. Samuel Friedman in New York City, Richard Rothenberg in Atlanta, Carl Latkin in Baltimore, and Robert Trotter in Flagstaff; each implemented, with their colleagues, network studies of their local populations at high risk for HIV infection, adapting our network survey instruments to their specific epidemiologic contexts. Each group produced notable results that advanced the science of applying the network framework to the epidemiology of sexually and parenterally (needles) transmissible infections.

Finally, it is gratifying to note that since the early 1990s there have been very few publications about the epidemiology of STD/HIV that have not referred to networks or/and to their probable impact on transmission of these infections. (Even the flagship American STD journal recently adopted network graphs as part of its permanent cover art, in January of 2012.) That is, arguably, the lasting contribution of our empirical work in Colorado Springs, for we showed that network assessment was feasible and provided strong evidence for the influence of network configuration on the propagation of several STD. For the Colorado Springs region, network analysis helped explain why, despite continued presence of high-risk behaviors, relatively little STD/HIV transmission seemed to be occurring.

SEVEN

WHY AFRICA? THE PUZZLE OF INTENSE HIV TRANSMISSION IN HETEROSEXUALS

This is a lean-forward, not a lean-back, chapter.

It is dedicated to Dr. Wallace Dinsmore,

unsung hero of this odyssey.

> "The philosophies of one age have become the
> absurdities of the next, and the foolishness of yesterday
> has become the wisdom of tomorrow."
> —Sir William Osler

Enter David Gisselquist, PhD a few months before my retirement

It started in the autumn of 2000 with a telephone call from Dr. David Gisselquist, a Yale-trained economist with an interest in the puzzle du jour: AIDS transmission in Africa. It seemed improbable to him that "heterosexual" transmission of HIV could be responsible for the turbocharged epidemics being reported from different parts of sub-Saharan Africa, principally from its eastern and southern regions. In perusing the literature in medical and public health journals, it struck him that the official version ascribing these intense epidemics to sexual intercourse was poorly supported by the available evidence. Besides, intense transmission of HIV in heterosexual populations *not engaging in injection of street drugs* was not being seen anywhere else in the world. So why Africa, which did not host large populations of injecting drug users? In the literature, he found a few articles by observers who doubted the official view espoused by the experts at the Centers For Disease Control (CDC) in Atlanta, the World Health Organization (WHO) in Geneva, and the recently formed agency in the United Nations (UNAIDS) also in Geneva. He contacted some of these skeptics,[1-6] one of whom was me. I told him that I was not very familiar with the HIV literature on sub-Saharan Africa, but suspected that use of unsterile needles in medical and ritualistic settings,[7] as well as local facilitating factors, such as tropical diseases that could damage the integrity of the tissues lining the genitals,[3] might be involved. He then asked if I would be interested in working on this problem with him; my reply was that I would be at greater leisure to do so after my retirement at the end of January 2001.

Our collaboration begins

As it was, Dr. Gisselquist had been doing a disciplined review of the literature on AIDS in Africa published during the previous twenty years, compiling and analyzing the evidence. His tack was to assess the quality and completeness of this evidence rather than to construct armchair arguments in speculative space, which was the most common approach to the question: "Why Africa?"

An outsider to the field of STD/HIV epidemiology, Dr. Gisselquist found it difficult to publish his findings in this field's professional journals. His first full-length article, which re-estimated the transmission efficiency of HIV through unsterilized medical injections, was rejected by three different journals during 2001.[8] Rejection slips for this and other manuscripts began to arrive at about the same time as my retirement. By then, I had also persuaded my long-term colleague Dr. Richard Rothenberg to assist in ameliorating Dr. Gisselquist's manuscripts for publication in medical journals. Working together and with other concerned observers, we published brief pieces (letters to the editor) in several medical journals calling attention to evidence inconsistent with the common view that sexual transmission could account for Africa's HIV epidemics.[9–13] As a newly (July 2000) minted member of the *International Journal of STD & AIDS'* editorial board, I knew that this journal would be interested in receiving quality manuscripts that other editors might reject, especially if these submissions did not necessarily echo the received wisdom. Both of Gisselquist's rejected full-length manuscripts, now edited and improved by experienced epidemiologists, were soon published by the *International Journal of STD & AIDS*.[8,14] These first letters and articles in 2002 marked the beginning of a long association between Dr. Gisselquist and me, along with several other colleagues who were to periodically contribute to subsequent manuscripts about AIDS in sub-Saharan Africa.

Impact of the early papers in the

International Journal of STD & AIDS

The second of Dr. Gisselquist's two full-length articles, co-authored by Drs. Rothenberg, Ernest Drucker and me, presented evidence from the literature showing large numbers of HIV infections in sub-Saharan Africa not explained by either sex or mother-to-child transmission.[14] This controversial paper challenged the official view that 90 percent of adult HIV cases in Africa had been contracted sexually; in Gisselquist's assessment[15] the official view was an assertion that had been decided without the facts, meaning a consensus was reached without the proper research to control for confound between sexual and non-sexual (skin puncturing) exposures. This 2002 paper was the one that triggered both furor and fury. It also stimulated the coalescing of an informal group calling for a new assessment of HIV transmission in Africa.[16] During the rest of the decade these skeptics, the majority of whom were not trained epidemiologists, were to produce dozens of publications questioning the received wisdom about AIDS transmission in Africa. The furor was the firestorm of commentary in the media and on the Internet; the fury was the angry reactions in the halls hosting the orthodox view: the CDC, the WHO, and UNAIDS. It turns out that this was a relatively mild dress rehearsal for the furor and fury triggered by publication of four additional papers in the same journal five months later.[17–20] The Royal Society of Medicine, publishers of the *International Journal of STD & AIDS*, soon responded to this attention by making this provocative article freely available, if only because the Society aimed to encourage debate.

Our earliest publications about sub-Saharan Africa's HIV epidemics,[8–9][14] all published in 2001–2002, provided converging evidence suggesting that much of HIV transmission could not be explained by sexual or mother-to-child transmission. The most glaring observation was that differences in sexual behaviors did not explain the different HIV epidemic trajectories on that continent. Although African hyper-sexuality was a time-honored stereotype in the western mind,[21] scientific sexual behavior surveys conducted during the late 1980s and early 1990s seriously damaged this stereotype by showing that reported levels of sexual activity (read: rates of partner change) in a dozen African countries[14] were comparable to those reported in European and North American surveys. These levels were *certainly* not greater by the order of magnitude difference needed to explain the turbocharged epidemics on that continent. Given that HIV transmission probabilities per penile-vaginal exposure in Africa had been shown to be similar to those observed in Europe and North America,[14] one would have to postulate not only greater rates of sexual partner change than studies were reporting but also phenomenal amounts of sexual activity for sex alone to account for observed levels of HIV infection in African adults.

In addition, studies contrasting the sexual behaviors of African adults living in areas of low- and high-prevalence showed little difference between these regions;[22] for example, the variables one would expect to

179

be related with sexual transmission of HIV, such as high rate of partner change, sex with prostitutes, sexually transmitted diseases, concurrent (as opposed to serial) sexual partnerships, dry sex (deliberately drying out the vagina to "tighten" it), and lack of condom use, were NOT more common in the high- versus low-prevalence regions. An intriguing observation was the *complete* disassociation in epidemic trajectories noted in Zimbabwe between STD and HIV during the 1990s: STD declined by 25% during that decade while HIV prevalence increased from 9% to 25%, implying a stunning 12% annual HIV increase.[13] Why would sets of sexually transmitted infections behave so differently during the same period in the same place unless modes of transmission other than simply sexual modes were involved? And why would a relatively low efficiency (in its sexual form of transmission) virus like HIV outrun the much more efficiently transmitted garden variety STD? Such data and considerations should have raised a red flag stimulating further epidemiologic investigation.

In addition, high rates of HIV infection were observed in very low-risk people: pregnant and post-partum women, especially women reporting only one lifetime sexual partner, with that partner having tested negative for HIV. Other low-risk people were the 10% or so of HIV-positive pre-pubertal children whose mothers had tested HIV-negative. Lastly, several studies had reported high levels of HIV infection associated with exposures to medical injections. For example: among factory workers in Rwanda in 1985, HIV prevalence in workers reporting a history of STD, but who had not received medical injections, was 9.7%, while those who had received medical injections had the significantly higher prevalence of 27%.[23] Altogether, such observations undermined the assertion that sex was responsible for virtually all HIV infections in African adults. (Officially, only a paltry 2% of infections were thought to be a consequence of non-sexual exposures by HIV-contaminated sharps.)

Defending the decided-without-the-facts consensus view

I was stunned by officialdom's response to this 2001–2002 set of publications critiquing the consensus view: in brief, they dug in their heels. Hard. Nor could I have begun to imagine that this initial response was to be their permanent response in the future, despite a cascade of subsequent publications that provided additional evidence to support this initial critique. The rational response would have been to admit that non-sexual exposures had been under-suspected for too long and had been scientifically under-explored. Programmatically, at the very least, there should have been a call to re-evaluate the evidence that led to the consensus in the first place, to assess its quality and reliability, and to field empiric studies to resolve dissonances— principally, to tease out the proportional contributions of sexual and non-sexual exposures to local HIV burdens.[24] This meant clearly accepting the fundamental fact that HIV was not a sexually transmitted, but a sexually *transmissible*, infection; there were far more effective ways other than sex to transmit it, and these ways should be properly investigated.

But this is not what happened. The mainstream view that sex was driving the HIV epidemics in sub-Saharan Africa was an assertion in dire need of high quality supportive evidence. Instead, as we shall see later, defenders principally relied on inferential reasoning and evidence of modest quality[25] to dismiss our arguments.[26] Reliance on such evidence to describe reality would have been tolerable had no anomalies or dissonances been observed. It is the breadth and depth of these dissonances that indicated the pressing need for a more rigorous look at HIV transmission dynamics in Africa. Our arguments were not only dismissed but, more importantly, ignored at the highest levels of the health agencies responsible for getting the picture right: CDC, WHO, and, especially, UNAIDS. Sadly, this silence at the highest levels continues to this day, despite more than a decade's worth of respectable evidence challenging the received wisdom.

Impact of the second wave of papers in the
International Journal of STD & AIDS

Five months after publication of our first full-length article on the topic[14] both furor and fury continued, but with greater intensity. What amplified the furor and fury was the simultaneous publication of four articles by our informal group in the March 2003 issue of the *International Journal of STD & AIDS*.[17–20] The Royal Society of Medicine orchestrated a press release on 20 February 2003 that received considerably more attention than the one four months prior, which had been based on a single article.[14] It is as if—to borrow a metaphor from the vaccination domain—the October press release primed the public, and the February one fully inoculated (not to be confused with "immunized") it.

Because Dr. Gisselquist's analyses tended to be exhaustively detailed and dryly reported, I designed and drafted the first article[17] of the series, focusing on presenting our arguments and evidence as simply and as straightforwardly as possible for both lay and professional readers. It summarized the dozen or so anomalies and dissonances, observing that the mounting toll of HIV infection in Africa echoed the mounting number of puzzling findings; in short, too many stubborn facts did not fit the official interpretation. The second article[18] presented, in ponderous detail, evidence that had been available in the refereed literature prior to promulgation of the consensus of 1988 by the WHO and the CDC. This evidence had either not been considered or had been inadequately interpreted. Not only did forging this official consensus represent a premature closing of debate about "Why Africa?" but it served to discourage further inquiry, not to mention dissent. By the time of the Fifth International Conference on AIDS in Montreal in mid-1989, for example, conversations and presentations about global HIV epidemiology failed to include consideration of non-sexual (blood-borne) HIV transmission in poor countries. That the consensus emerged despite, rather than from, the available evidence did not speak highly for the scientific trustworthiness of the public health bureaucracies charged with the serious task of getting the epidemiologic picture right. A good part of the reason for this official failure is the well-known tendency of experts to ignore evidence they do not want to see especially, I suspect, if such evidence could jeopardize funding streams. Both considerations can discourage implementation of properly controlled and conducted field studies, for fear that results might not only undermine the experts' cherished views but also their livelihood.

By detailing the evidence that had appeared in the literature prior to the official forging of the consensus, which averred that the vast majority of HIV cases in sub-Saharan Africa were the result of unprotected sex, our informal group managed to trigger the fury of many at the WHO, the CDC, and UNAIDS. I speculate that offended members of these health organizations viewed our analysis as an unkind assessment of their scientific competence or, perhaps, of their political-ideological motives (more on that later). I was very surprised at their reaction because I naively thought that they would be considerate of our suggestion, based on very good evidence, that the problem of anomalies and dissonances could be solved by comprehensively evaluating the contribution of non-sexual modes of transmission to HIV burdens in poor countries. I could not have been more wrong. They reacted with shock, dismay, and anger. And, as we will soon see, their response mainly consisted of rationalizing away the dissonances within the framework of the orthodoxy. In brief, they used their belief framework as a substitute for better evidence.

Just what did this pre-1988 consensus evidence suggest? It could actually best be used to support the interpretation that health care exposures in Africa caused more HIV infections than sexual transmission! This was a stunning realization. Note that I did not say "revelation", for this would require data from really well-designed studies. After all, extraordinary claims require extraordinary evidence. In any event, the admittedly crude measures of risk factors obtained from published study samples of the general population were shown to associate more than half of HIV infections in adults with puncturing exposures in health care settings.[18] But that wasn't all. Gisselquist also used these data to construct a mathematical model designed to estimate the proportion of HIV in Africa that was caused by sex;[19] the model indicated that only about 25%–29% of HIV incidence in African women, and about 30%–35% in men, could be attributed to sexual exposures. True, the substandard quality of the data emanating from Africa and the generally poorly designed research studies prevented us from making definitive statements. As we concluded,[19] "We cannot and do not intend our estimates to be the last word, but rather a step toward better evidence-based estimates…"

Our last article in this controversial issue of the *International Journal of STD & AIDS*[20] critiqued the claim that improved management of sexually transmitted diseases in Mwanza, Tanzania during the early 1990s had subsequently caused a nearly 40 percent decline in new HIV infections. This result was suspicious because, while the incidence of HIV infection had dramatically (minus 38%) declined, the garden-variety STD burden had not. Moreover, the researchers had not controlled for the contemporaneous implementation of sterile health care protocols and training in Mwanzan clinics by a different public health team.[27] Our article called for re-analysis of the Mwanza trial data in light of these considerations. This was not done or, if done, it was not reported.

Analyses and reflections in these four simultaneously published papers should have injected enough doubt in the minds of experts that research agendas should have been re-conceptualized and modified accordingly. This was not to be. Shockingly, refusal to properly investigate non-sexual HIV transmission modes remains true as of the date of this writing (Spring 2015): reported studies controlling for these kinds of confounding factors are exceedingly rare. And I certainly did not endear myself to the CDC, WHO, and UNAIDS experts when I told them, behind closed doors on 14 March 2003, that HIV epidemiology in sub-Saharan Africa consisted of "First World researchers doing second rate science in Third World countries." But it was and remains true. When all is said and done, what kind of science is it that ignores a potentially major mode of transmission by obstinately refusing to properly measure it?

"I and my public understand each other very well; it doesn't hear what I say, and I don't say what it wants to hear."

—Karl Kraus

From here to enmity: the March 14, 2003 meeting in Geneva

The international health agencies' formal response to our controversial papers was to convene a meeting of experts at WHO headquarters in Geneva shortly after these articles' appearance in print. The idea, as stated in the memorandum to participants, was to "bring together the leading epidemiological and modeling experts with Gisselquist and Potterat" and to "prepare the ground for a strong well founded statement from WHO and UNAIDS on the role of unsafe injections in HIV transmission. This statement will have to be published in a leading scientific journal, and also has to be disseminated widely in the press. There will not be a report from the meeting itself."[28] Regrettably, this meeting was neither tape- nor video-recorded. There were approximately thirty participants, including at least five from WHO, two each from UNAIDS and CDC, five from European schools of tropical medicine, one each from the National Institute of Allergy and Infectious Diseases, the US Agency for International Development, and Immunization, and three of us (Drs. Stuart Brody, David Gisselquist, and me).

It turns out that this "consultation" was to set the tone for all subsequent discourse about what was driving HIV transmission in poor countries. First, no one from the highest echelons of the three international health agencies was present at this consultation, foreshadowing their future and continuing absence from public commentary on this discussion, in either the media or in the scientific literature, other than the occasional pro forma denial that anything but sex could be responsible for HIV epidemics in Africa. Second, their official response was highly choreographed, bureaucratic (read: science by committee), and dismissive of the evidence and arguments presented. The orthodoxy was staunchly reaffirmed and continued to be buttressed by weak empiric evidence—although the conclusion was capped by a (soon to prove hollow) promise to obtain "improved data"[26] to strengthen confidence in the mainstream view. Third, the free-floating anger that was part of the background noise at the meeting, and which several times flared into ill-tempered remarks, was to remain part of the subsequent discourse.

The press release summarizing the proceedings not only misrepresented the sense and outcome of the consultation but it was finalized *before* the end of the deliberations. It therefore became clear to us that the international agencies' minds were made up before the meeting. What was reported was that although "no consensus emerged from the conference", the "prevailing view was that sexual transmission was responsible for the large majority of HIV infections in sub-Saharan Africa; *Gisselquist and colleagues demurred* (Emphasis mine)." This was "prevailing view" by plebiscite: there were many more persons present at that meeting supporting the orthodoxy than those questioning it or *willing to voice skepticism*. What the press release *should* have emphasized is that the studies cited during the discussions by participants committed to the orthodox view at best provided only weak support for that view. Indeed, lack of evidence supporting the orthodox view *was why the press release concluded with a call for better data* to more definitively determine the role of puncturing exposures in HIV transmission.

And yet "better data" were already available but conveniently ignored. One of the experts at this March 2003 meeting presented unpublished data from Uganda showing incident (new cases) HIV to be more common among people reporting medical injections than among those who didn't. These data were eventually published, but 4 years later.[29] Moreover, the CDC had recently reviewed a UNAIDS-commissioned research study by one of its own which showed that there was a strong "association between HIV infection and health care injections. Incidence studies, all conducted in sub-Saharan Africa, indicated that contaminated injections may cause between 12% and 33% of new infections in the region."[30] The paper, reviewed in Atlanta in the early autumn of 2002, was not cleared for publication by the international health agencies (CDC, WHO, and UNAIDS).

For me, the singular memory I retain from this long ago meeting was the comment made to us by a ranking and seasoned representative of an internationally respected health agency that "maybe you're right [about puncturing exposures] but don't tell the African people". I was stunned. This was spontaneously (?) uttered, presumably because this kind of information could jeopardize public health initiatives such as vaccination campaigns—as if Africans were not smart enough to pay attention to two different risks at once. That person also said "I cannot wrap my mind around this". I now certainly knew who wasn't smart enough to understand, and it wasn't African adults.

A distillation of these proceedings, which omitted the evidence presented at the meeting that was unsupportive of the orthodoxy, appeared in the high-impact medical journal, *The Lancet*, one year later.[26] This influential article, spearheaded by the WHO, concluded that "there is no compelling evidence that unsafe injections are a predominant mode of HIV-1 transmission in sub-Saharan Africa". Crucially, it failed to address the key anomalies that indicated that sex was not the main driver of the epidemics in Africa. Yet its anemic rebuttal of our analyses effectively closed the door to more rigorous inspection of transmission dynamics in Africa. Indeed, it continues to be the article customarily cited in support of the orthodoxy and invoked to dismiss dissenting views such as ours.

Here is not the place to detail the arguments and evidence the international agencies presented to rebut us, but to emphasize that they focused narrowly on medical injections in formal health care settings, rather than also considering other forms of puncturing exposures, such as phlebotomy (blood testing) and exposures in informal health care and ritualistic (for example, tattooing) settings. Moreover, they ignored their own research when it supported our position.[29–30] As for manner, they relied principally on ecologic evidence, which is the most distant from the actual transmission events and settings,[31] on risk factor evidence derived from inadequate (read: uncontrolled for puncturing exposures and proper measures of anal intercourse) studies; on inferential reasoning; on speculation; and what they consider to be logical rather than relying on quality data.

Their counter arguments also relied on wholesale rejection of the evidence we presented, claiming that many findings were not true because patients had lied about their sex lives; because mistakes had been made in HIV testing procedures; and because the data were too old and, by insinuation, untrustworthy. In brief: they selectively denied the validity of the evidence they did not like. When in doubt, blame the data. In my opinion, they chose not to believe the evidence because they did not want to. In any event, their position reminded me of the famous line uttered by the professor in Alfred Hitchcock's movie *The Lady Vanishes*: "Nonsense, my theory is perfectly correct. It is the facts that are misleading." And that, in a nutshell, summarizes the official countering of our analyses.

Exiting the consultation meeting at WHO headquarters late that Friday afternoon, Dr. Brody and I entered the elevator. By (what we thought might be) good luck, its occupant was the WHO Secretary General, accompanied by an armed bodyguard. Noticing our meeting identification badges, she mentioned that she had been informed that a consensus had been reached at this consultation. Dr. Brody assured her that not only was this not the case, but that the "consensus" statement had been decided, and even disseminated, before the meeting was over. At that point, the elevator reached the bottom floor and we all exited with polite "good evenings". Two days later, after our return home, Dr. Brody, Dr. Gisselquist and I emailed the Secretary General, reminding her of our recent encounter in the elevator, and reiterating that the WHO press release "misrepresented both the sense and the outcome of the consultation"; we requested that the inaccurate press release be rescinded and offered our assistance "in the drafting of an accurate consensus statement". She never replied.

The U.S. Congress reacts

Our papers' conclusions also reached the ears of Congress. Under the leadership of Senator Jeff Sessions (R-Alabama), the US Senate Committee on Health, Education, Labor, and Pensions held hearings shortly after publication of our four articles, to determine whether HIV/AIDS funds should be earmarked for programs targeting unsafe puncturing exposures. (Sessions's staff had contacted Dr. Gisselquist and me almost immediately, on 10 March 2003.) Senator Sessions, via the Department of Health and Human Services, also commissioned RTI International, an independent and non-profit research institution, to assess our claims that contaminated needles might well be driving the HIV epidemics in sub-Saharan Africa. The RTI report,[32] released in early January 2004, concluded that "Arguments used to inform the debate about the etiologic significance of unsafe medical injections for HIV infection in sub-Saharan Africa or the Caribbean are based on meager evidence at best." (Ironically, the same criticism could much more fairly be applied to the assertion that heterosexual sex was driving the epidemics!) Importantly, the report noted the inadequacies in the published literature, principally the lack of quality and relevant studies to confidently settle the issue. The report (properly) recommended that unpublished data that could shed light on the issue *should be solicited* and published, and that *new, well-designed studies be implemented* as indicated. Neither recommendation, to my knowledge, was ever followed. The report also concluded that, until shown to be misdirected, HIV control efforts in Africa should stay the course. This was, to me, the equivalent of temporarily settling the issue using an epidemiologic penalty shoot-out. In any event, at least Senator Sessions was able through two hearings to generate support to target $300 million out of the President's Emergency Program for AIDS Relief (PEPFAR), primarily in Africa, to promote safe injections and safe blood transfusions.

"I believe in getting into hot water. I think it keeps you clean."

—G. K. Chesterton

Explaining the resistance to our critique and reflections

Skepticism disturbs orthodoxy. Predictably, doubting often produces defensive reactions from believers, ranging from irritation to rage.[33] Defensiveness on the part of the international health agencies and mainstream HIV researchers was strong, far stronger than any of us had anticipated. It was closer to the rage, than irritation, end of the spectrum. Nor had we anticipated that part of their reaction would include (unflattering) ad hominem comments. Among other, less printable, things I was called "Africa's Newest Plague"; "Core

Stigmatizer"; "Linus Pauling—in his later years" (when Pauling was thought to be advancing crackpot ideas); and [a reward being offered] "for his head on a platter". There may come a time in one's professional life when one loses respect for colleagues once admired. These adrenal cortex-derived epithets were *my* baptism under fire, because each of them emanated from esteemed colleagues in these agencies; they were uncalled for, considering that the only thing I stigmatized was shoddy science, that predictable impostor of truth.

By their own admission, the international agencies feared that our work would cause Africans to lose trust in modern health care, especially childhood immunizations, as well as undermine safer sex initiatives. (Recall that their condom campaigns were also aimed at curtailing rapid population growth in sub-Saharan Africa.) We *speculate* that disbelief on the part of HIV researchers that medical care in Africa could be harming patients may have been a significant factor in their defensive posture. We were also impugning the quality of their scientific research and potentially threatening their livelihoods. In addition, our analyses also directly threatened the politically correct view that AIDS was not just a disease of gay men and injecting drug users, but also of heterosexuals. Lastly, our data were undermining the time-honored belief about African promiscuity, a notion that may well have initially contributed to the (pre)conception that AIDS was thriving in Africa because of it.

"God was satisfied with his own work, and that is fatal."

—Samuel Butler

The aftermath

The international health agencies and mainstream HIV-in-Africa researchers essentially stonewalled our views by denigrating, dismissing, or ignoring the evidence we were presenting—all the while asserting, ex cathedra, that their catechism was right. The few who (semi-)publicly reserved judgment until better evidence arrived soon became silent, not only because better evidence in the form of well-designed studies had not been forthcoming but because, gauging the ferocity of the resistance, they probably succumbed to peer pressure and chose to remain on the sidelines, whatever their private views might have been.

Two attributes color the study of HIV transmission in Africa: lack of tolerance for dissent and, above all, virtual absence of publicly expressed skepticism for the orthodoxy in the halls of mainstream public health organizations and of academia. Received wisdom, uncritically accepted, usually ossifies into dogma. This is precisely what happened. Regrettably, lack of tolerance soon reached the editorial offices of the major medical and public health journals. We *speculate* that the international health agencies and mainstream reviewers persuaded the editorial staffs at these high-impact journals not to publish our papers, probably by asserting that our views would be detrimental to HIV interventions in Africa and would contribute to increases in HIV

195

transmissions and mortality. In this regard it was truly unfortunate that AIDS deniers like the Duesbergians[34] had previously given dissent a bad name. Whereas Duesbergians denied that HIV caused AIDS, we knew that the evidence for HIV causing AIDS was incontrovertible and said so. Yet somehow we seemingly were lumped with the Duesbergians and other deniers.[34] As I specifically pointed out elsewhere, there is a world of difference between dissenters, which we are, and deniers, which we are not.[35]

Post Geneva meeting publications: manner

During the ten years following the Geneva "consultation" we publicly[36] encouraged both debate of available evidence and implementation of well-designed studies, and this was a frequent part of the concluding remarks of our publications. Our informal group, whose membership fluctuated during this period, eventually published dozens of full-length articles, commentaries, and letters to the editor. After a series of rejections from top journals, we lowered our expectations and generally submitted manuscripts to lower-impact journals. Of the 55 original articles (and 6 commentaries) eventually published, 34 (56%) appeared in the *International Journal of STD & AIDS*. (This apparent favoritism was probably the major reason for sacking the editor-in-chief, Dr. Wallace Dinsmore—a founding editor of the journal—in early 2010 after 20 years at the helm.) We were also inveterate scientific correspondents, sending 82 letters about AIDS in Africa to editors of medical and public health journals, 55 (67%) of which were published

(See Appendix 2). Of the unpublished letters, almost all were rejected by high-impact American journals such as *Science* and the *Journal of the American Medical Association*. It is a tribute to editors of several British medical journals that they were much more willing to publish our articles, editorials, and letters than journals elsewhere. *Indeed it is astonishing that virtually no scholarly debate on the controversy surrounding HIV transmissions in Africa took place within the pages of American medical or public health journals.*

Post Geneva meeting publications: matter

Our informal group's post Geneva meeting publications focused on 1) providing more evidence suggestive of the importance of non-sexual HIV transmission in sub-Saharan Africa (full-length articles) and 2) critiquing newly published studies, pointing out errors of commission and omission, and suggesting ways to achieve adequate data analysis and/or offering more logic- and evidence-driven interpretations of their data (letters to the editor) and 3) providing commentary (editorials).

For example, one of the objections by the international agencies to our suggestions that non-sexual (puncturing) exposures might be driving the HIV epidemics was the apparent absence of HIV in children ages 5 to 12. They argued that were such exposures common, children would be as much at risk as adults. Actually this was a largely data-free inference. Children were unlikely to be medically attended at (say) prenatal or STD clinics, where HIV prevalence was known to be very high; hence their exposure risk would be different from that of adults attending such clinics. Secondly, surveys of HIV prevalence in pediatric populations had rarely been conducted. In several articles we discussed the implications of a then recent national probability sample of the South African population showing an astonishing HIV positivity rate of 5.6% for 5–12 year olds.[37] Their reply was that the testing had been faulty, again blaming the data. In a series of later publications, we showed that this result was not an anomaly.[38–44] We summarized dozens of prior studies of pediatric HIV infection in clinical settings; these reported young children becoming infected from sources other than their (uninfected) mothers.[39] We published analyses of alarmingly high rates of HIV in young children in Mozambique,[43] Swaziland,[41] Kenya,[41] and Uganda[44] based (mostly) on independently conducted nationally representative surveys in these countries. In light of such findings, the proper response would have been to conduct surveys in several different countries with high and low HIV prevalence, making sure that testing protocols and specimen processing were scientifically unimpeachable—using cases and controls, contact tracing, comprehensive assessment of risks, and sequencing ("fingerprinting") of HIV. None of this was done.

Another objection on the part of the international health agencies was that we had grossly overestimated the efficiency of HIV transmission under various skin puncturing circumstances. This putative "overestimate" had allowed them to reject our claims out of hand. We therefore conducted an extensive review of available data in the medical literature [45] concluding that *their* assessment was probably wrong by an order of magnitude. Yet, aware that our data were incomplete, we admitted that our conclusion was in need of improved data via new studies. To my knowledge, such studies have not been fielded.

A particularly damaging article appeared in the prestigious journal *Nature* in the form of a brief communication in 2003. It concluded that, because HIV and Hepatitis-C prevalence patterns in sub-Saharan Africa do not often coincide, puncturing exposures were "not the dominant contributor to the African epidemic".[46] Actually, this ecologic inference was faulty, as we detailed in a rebuttal shortly afterward, but in a different venue.[47] (Nature declined to publish our rebuttal.) The principal weakness of their argument was the assumption that these two different blood-borne viruses were transmitted the same way In fact, Hepatitis-C was known to be efficiently transmitted *intravenously* (into the veins) but not *intramuscularly* (usual route for medical injections)—therefore, a different epidemic pattern could be *expected*. In addition, the prevalence data they used to plot Hepatitis-C patterns were based on old and unrepresentative surveys, not to mention that tests for Hepatitis-C were often insensitive to detecting African strains, as a recently (2015) reported study confirmed.[48] In the intervening decade, however, no studies had been fielded to resolve these uncertainties.

We also published articles indicating that anal intercourse in heterosexual African populations was likely to be more common than currently believed, and we suggested ways to obtain valid research results.[49–52] Regrettably, this did not result in modification of prevention messages to specifically address the dangers of anal intercourse. In addition, we published results of analyses showing that HIV infection was much more common in circumcised than in uncircumcised virgins of either sex and in adolescents in Kenya, Lesotho, and South Africa, implicating non-sexual transmission.[53] Moreover, our collaborators published several analyses highly suggestive of HIV transmission in medical settings[54–57] and what could be done to attenuate such risks.[58] In this regard, we proposed that several policies could be *immediately and inexpensively* implemented: 1) broad public education about non-sexual risks; 2) transparent (patient-observed) sterile medical care procedures; and 3) zero tolerance for health care associated infections.[58] We recommended implementation of quality control in health care settings and, crucially, investigation of unexplained HIV infections; both of these aspects of health care delivery were routinely conducted in rich countries and should be supported in poor countries as a priority.[59]

Only when people have accurate knowledge of HIV modes of transmission can they make good decisions to protect themselves and their families from inadvertent infection. Hence the importance of public education. Dr. Devon Brewer tested this view and attempted to measure its impact by examining Demographic and Health Survey data from 16 sub-Saharan African countries.[60] In a cleverly thought out analysis, he concentrated on examining data that could illuminate his question: is knowledge of *blood-borne* (not sexual, which everybody in Africa knows about) HIV risk associated with a country's HIV prevalence? It turned out that countries in which many people were aware of blood-borne risk indeed had lower HIV prevalence than countries in which few people were aware of such risk. This observation suggests that explicit public education campaigns about *blood-borne* (read: puncturing exposures) HIV risk may be very important in protecting the population from such exposures.

The narrow focus on sexual transmission of HIV can lead to deeply harmful and unwarranted stigma, such as for an infected woman whose sole lifetime sexual partner is her HIV-negative husband. We specifically addressed this danger in a commentary.[61] It is the default assumption of sexual transmission that puts such infected women in the position of being unfairly accused of infidelity or promiscuity. Silence about non-sexual exposures destroys reputations and lives, with women in traditional African societies being particularly vulnerable to abuse and abandonment.[61]

Countering UNAIDS/WHO/CDC inertia and inaction

By mid-decade, it was clear that the dozens of publications presenting evidence undermining the official view that heterosexual transmission was driving sub-Saharan Africa's epidemics had failed to have the intended impact of stimulating scientifically sound research. As we had previously pointed out, what was needed was evidence that one could have confidence in. Because we were unaware of any research being done to do the required studies and because we despaired that these would ever be done in our lifetime, Dr. Brewer suggested we do our own. This was a bold suggestion, considering that we not only lived a long way from Africa, but also had no source of funding. We also knew that grant proposal reviewers, being affiliated with the international health agencies or with the preponderantly scientifically conservative academia, would be unlikely to approve our proposals should we apply. What is viewed as maverick science has a predictably tough time being funded.

Luckily, some members of our informal group had contacts on the ground in Africa. For example, Dr. Gisselquist's other field of expertise, agricultural policy, frequently engaged him as a consultant in both South Asia and sub-Saharan Africa, while Dr. Brewer's interest in assessing blood exposures in non-formal health settings (viz., traditional medical practitioners) led him to contact the author of an article on such risks in *Tropical Doctor*[62]—a Nigerian physician practicing in a teaching hospital in Calabar, located in the southeastern coastal region of the country. Dr. Gisselquist's connection, an enterprising part-time journalist from Kenya named Moses Okinyi and Dr. Brewer's connection, Dr. Etete Peters, were both willing to participate in our efforts to implement two empiric studies, one involving HIV-infected children in Kenya and the other, involving newly infected adults in Nigeria.

2007: A turning point year—or so we hoped.

After at least five years of providing evidence that the mainstream view ought to be reconsidered, a recommendation that fell on unwilling if not deaf, ears, Dr. Gisselquist decided to publish a book summarizing our findings and make it freely available on the internet,[59] bearing the felicitous double-entendre title of "Points to Consider...". Contemporaneously, Dr. Brewer and I decided to field 2 studies on the ground in Africa, despite lack of outside funding. It was hoped that Gisselquist's book would attract the attention of thoughtful persons outside the entrenched AIDS industry and thus maybe bring pressure on the AIDS-in-Africa establishment to do what was scientifically correct. This apparently did not happen.

The first field study was carried out in Calabar, Nigeria between August 2007 and February 2008, under the aegis of Dr. Etete Peters and his medical students. Because we had long thought about proper study design to assess the contribution of sexual and non-sexual exposures, we took the lead in proposing a survey instrument that would prospectively and comprehensively assess both sexual and non-sexual (puncturing) exposures in newly-infected patients in Dr. Peters's clinics. This survey instrument's architect was Dr. Brewer who collegially solicited suggestions from his American and African collaborators. Dr. Brewer was especially interested in controlling for "reverse causation" because this had been one of the main objections by mainstream researchers to our evidence that medical procedures were driving HIV epidemics in Africa. "Reverse causation" refers to misinterpreting the sometimes strong association between, say, medical injections and HIV prevalence by concluding that HIV-infected patients had become infected while attending a clinic for medical care when, in point of fact, it could be that these HIV-infected patients had been previously infected (by sex, naturally!) and were attending a clinic because they were now sick with symptoms of advanced HIV infection. Hence an important aim of the study was "to assess the relationship between a broad array of blood exposures, especially those not received in response to HIV-related symptoms or complications, and incident HIV infection in sub-Saharan Africa".[63]

The study's participants were recruited from the voluntary HIV testing clinics at the University of Calabar's Teaching Hospital. About three-quarters of clients approached were successfully enrolled; remarkably, most declined the approximately $5 compensation offered to cover transportation costs. During the six-month study interval, 321 clients participated. Because our interest was HIV incidence, analyses focused on serial testers: with them, one could observe the change from last negative test to first positive test. Forty-five clients were serial testers, of whom 10 became HIV infected during the study period, for a (high) 10% annual incidence rate. In brief, although we found that many types of blood exposures were commonly reported, persons who became HIV-infected were more likely to report both specific and aggregate blood exposures during the study period than persons who remained uninfected. Crucially, newly HIV-infected clients reported blood exposures that could not be explained to be a consequence of seeking medical care for symptoms of HIV, thereby undermining mainstream researchers' conviction that reverse causation accounted for the association between medical care and HIV prevalence. Nor could newly-acquired HIV infection be accounted for by unprotected sexual exposures: no sexual variable was associated with newly-acquired HIV infection. HIV incident cases were associated with use of someone else's razor, surgery, blood transfusions, enemas, vaccinations, and infusions. The principal shortcoming of this study was the small number of serial testers and of incident cases (ten). Yet this pilot study supported our contentions and should have provoked the conducting of larger studies to confirm our findings.[63] Regrettably, this did not happen.

The second field study was also initiated in 2007 and lasted one year, starting in March.[41] Like the first, it was a case-control study, but took place in Kenya, and focused on HIV-infected children rather than adults. These children had HIV-negative mothers and, therefore, were not likely to have acquired infection at birth or while their mother breast-fed them. As in the Nigerian case-control study, these HIV-infected patients, whose controls were their own HIV-negative siblings, were shown to have had more kinds of blood exposures than their uninfected siblings. In particular, punctures related to health care for malaria (blood testing, injections, infusions), and dental surgery by informal providers, were more commonly reported in HIV-infected children, confirming previous findings in a South African pediatric survey[37]—the same one that the WHO had denigrated by blaming the data's quality. We also combined these Kenyan findings with those of a representative national health survey in Swaziland conducted between 2006 and 2007 that included 1665 children aged 2 to 12. Fifty Swazi children (3%) in the sample were HIV-positive, with 11 (22%) of the 50 having HIV-negative mothers.[41] From this observation, we inferred that 1808 children aged 2 to 12 in Swaziland had HIV and HIV-negative mothers, implying infection by some non-sexual means, possibly contaminated sharps (because infection via the sexual route, including sexual abuse, was deemed very unlikely). Although the Swazi press rapidly disseminated our findings[64] and although this publicity prompted a public call for investigation by a Swazi Crown Prince, interest quickly fizzled and no follow-up was, to our knowledge, ever done by Swazi authorities. And, unsurprisingly, no follow-up studies or investigations were done by mainstream researchers or by international health agencies to challenge or confirm these findings, or to protect other children via finding the source of these unexplained infections. And it's not as if these would have been expensive studies to implement: I personally funded the two studies[41,63] for less than 10,000 US dollars. All things considered, 2007 was not a turning point year. Sigh.

Other voices

Between 2006 and 2014, several studies appeared in the literature whose empiric results were supportive of our view that HIV transmission dynamics in sub-Saharan Africa seriously needed revisiting. Among them, one of the most persuasive was done by the CDC's own Dr. Janet St. Lawrence and her colleagues,[65] who had historical (1989–2001) risk factor data on more than 3000 pregnant women at University Teaching Hospital in Lusaka, Zambia. These women were about 24 years old, married (90%) and monogamous (90% with no other partner in the previous three years), yet an astonishing thirty percent were HIV-infected. Not only were injections, both intramuscular and intravenous, overwhelmingly associated with HIV infection in these women—far exceeding the contribution of sexual behaviors—but HIV infection could clearly not be blamed on reverse causation. Only 4 of the 11 sexual behaviors measured were associated with HIV infection, yet, counter-intuitively, they were *inversely* associated, implying that sexual behaviors were protective of HIV infection! Clearly such findings should have triggered flashing red lights. On the contrary, this retrospective study so upset the CDC that Dr. St Lawrence was asked not to publish it. She refused her superiors' request. Turned down by several high-impact journals, the manuscript was eventually submitted, at my recommendation, to the *International Journal of STD & AIDS*. Once peer-reviewed and accepted for publication, the CDC pressured its editor-in-chief, Dr. Dinsmore, and publisher (the Royal Society of Medicine) to withdraw acceptance. Dr.

Dinsmore's courageous decision to publish it anyway saved this important analysis from disappearing into medical oblivion, as happened with a previous CDC study mentioned earlier.[30] Dr. St. Lawrence was due to retire from the CDC shortly afterward and she (understandably) opted to do so.

Another investigator whose analyses made it foolish to ignore or dismiss findings suggestive of a substantial role for puncturing exposures in sub-Saharan Africa's HIV epidemics was Savanna Reid. She and her colleague van Niekerk used information from official South African surveys to conclude that omission of non-sexual transmission from consensus HIV epidemiology in Africa was not only a serious oversight, but had profound ethical and operational implications for interventions.[66] Among other findings, they pointed out that more than a quarter of recent HIV infections detected in the 2005 South African national survey occurred in adults who denied sex during the previous twelve months; they presented evidence showing that only a very high rate of misreporting could produce this stunning observation—this particular comment aimed at readers inclined to dismiss this finding by saying that participants had lied about their sex lives. They also reported on recent surveys that indicated widespread lapses in infection control in health and dental care facilities,[67] subverting the commonly held view that medical care in South Africa was of high quality and safe.[26]

Moreover, Reid undermined the assertion by mainstream researchers that if injections were driving the HIV epidemics, one would see many more HIV-infected kids aged 2 to 12 years.[40] She challenged it with a meta-analysis of published literature and with mathematical modeling to indicate that HIV prevalence in children would not likely increase with age, as mainstream researchers had insisted. Here, then, was yet another petard under a mainstream assumption that had not, in the first place, been supported by data, only by inference and speculation. In addition, Reid and another colleague (Juma) independently estimated the risk of HIV transmission during blood exposures taking both viral and host characteristics into account, concluding that three separate avenues of evidence (infective dose, viral load, and injection volume) support Gisselquist's estimates that HIV transmission efficiency is likely to be considerably higher than that believed by mainstream HIV researchers.[68] Finally, Reid pointed out a serious error in the WHO estimates[69] that contaminated injections accounted for only 2.5% of HIV infections in sub-Saharan Africa. The error consisted of the WHO model having used the general population's rate of HIV prevalence rather than the more relevant HIV prevalence in clinics to calculate frequency of exposure to contaminated injections; this would be especially important in clinics seeing patients experiencing advanced disease, which is known to be more infectious than latent infection. Reid's model adjustments raised the estimated contribution by medical injections from 2.5% to somewhere between 12% and 47%, a considerable difference.[69]

By mid-decade, my long-time colleague Stuart Brody had been contacted by a German graduate student, Eva Deuchert, to help assess available data on health care in Africa that made little sense to her. In several papers, she and Brody provided additional evidence suggestive of an important role for health care related HIV transmission.[54–57] The first paper showed that Kenyan women who received tetanus shots during pregnancy were about twice as likely to have HIV infection compared to women who had not received this vaccination.[54] Importantly, these findings were not confounded by reverse causality; not only were tetanus shots prophylactic rather than given for treatment for disease symptoms, but none of the infected women was even aware that she had HIV infection. The second paper showed that specific health care indicators (for example, failure to use disposable syringes designed to only be used once, and broader implementation of tetanus vaccination) were strongly associated with HIV prevalence in African countries with available data.[57] The third, and highly technical, paper[55] showed that mathematical models generally used to simulate heterosexual HIV epidemics suffer from use of model parameters that are distant from evidence on the ground. Hence simulations have not accurately portrayed the epidemics in sub-Saharan Africa. The authors detail how many models have used grossly inflated per-contact HIV transmission probabilities, grossly overestimate numbers of sexual partners African adults have, and grossly overestimate frequency of their sexual activity.

Starting mid-decade, several other investigators outside our informal group began reporting findings that undermined the mainstream orthodoxy that sex was driving HIV epidemics in Africa. First, a little detour. In the early days, it was widely accepted in both policy and scholarly circles that sexual promiscuity explained "Why Africa?" When population-based surveys, conducted during the late 1980s/early 1990s, failed to support the idea of African hyper-sexuality,[14] researchers speculated that sexual concurrency (overlapping partners instead of serial partnering) accounted for the extraordinarily rapid rates of HIV infection, particularly in eastern and southern Africa. Although the renowned Four-Cities study[22] at the beginning of the new millennium, and our own observations a year later,[11] provided persuasive evidence that sexual concurrency was not likely to explain "Why Africa?", defenders of this notion were undaunted and *shrilly* continued to advocate its importance. Helen Epstein, for example, wrote a widely publicized book half a decade later claiming that discouraging long term concurrency could be Africa's "invisible cure".[70] As I stated elsewhere, this was clearly a case of "invisible evidence".[71] Two years later, Lurie and Rosenthal published a landmark analysis[72] showing that there was not any conclusive evidence in Africa that concurrency was associated with HIV prevalence or with increases in the size of the HIV epidemics or with increases in the speed of HIV transmission or with HIV persistence in populations. Shortly thereafter, Sawers and Stillwaggon meticulously examined the concurrency mathematical model—warts and all—and its unrealistic (their word) assumptions and came to a similar conclusion: there is no correlation between sexual

211

concurrency and HIV prevalence in Africa.[73] The warts? In their own words: "…quantitative evidence cited by proponents of the concurrency hypothesis is unconvincing since they exclude Demographic and Health Surveys and other data showing that concurrency in Africa is low, make broad statements about non-African concurrency based on very few surveys, report data incorrectly, report data from studies that have no information about concurrency as though they supported the hypothesis, report incomparable data and cite unpublished or unavailable studies."[73] This damning scholarly assessment could easily be the template for most of the mainstream HIV epidemiology research in Africa.

Sawers and Stillwaggon, along with Hertz, also provided evidence for HIV transmission-boosting factors that have been neglected by mainstream researchers: "endemic parasitic and infectious diseases… [that] increase the likelihood of HIV infection and alter the dynamics of epidemic spread."[74] They present data from many developing countries that diseases such as schistosomiasis, lymphatic filariasis, gonorrhea, chlamydia and malaria, for example, may well be the transmission-boosting co-factors that could explain "Why Africa?" In any event, these authors state that business-as-usual-sex-behavior-driven epidemiology needs to be given a permanent rest, since it has so consistently and so long failed to solve this puzzle.

Akeke and colleagues[75] reported on how frequently inmates in a Lesotho prison, 90% of whom are in the high-risk years for HIV, received tattoos while in detention: two-thirds of the nearly half who sported tattoos. They note that tattooing instruments in prisons were seldom sterilized and, half of the time, were used serially on several inmates. Although no HIV results were reported, this African report echoed one from the previous year in Georgia (USA) that noted a strong association between receiving a tattoo in prison and HIV incidence in inmates.[76] These observations clearly suggested the need for a closer look at tattooing as a probable contributor to HIV transmission in Africa.

Apetrei and colleagues investigated the risk of HIV transmission through unsafe injections.[77] Not only had this transmission route been asserted by mainstream epidemiologists to be, in the absence of convincing evidence, too inefficient to contribute significantly to Africa's HIV epidemics,[26] but two papers published the following year had buttressed that assertion. An investigation in Ethiopia, using suboptimal laboratory techniques, had failed to find HIV in needles that had been used on clinic patients in areas the authors claimed—without providing data—to have high HIV prevalence.[78] Another study, conducted in Zimbabwe, specifically excluded unsafe injections as a major source of HIV in that country.[79] Apetrei's group, using rigorous laboratory techniques, demonstrated that HIV was present in 33% of syringes used for *intravenous* injections and in 2.3% of syringes used for *intramuscular* injections.[77] As the authors conclude: "…we provided proof of concept that injection practices could account for a significant proportion of new HIV infections." The different findings from these three African countries should have prompted the launching of other studies to settle this important issue. This did not happen.

Lastly, two of the most seasoned epidemiologists working in sub-Saharan Africa recently admitted: "We still do not fully understand why the spread of HIV has been (and still is) so different in sub-Saharan Africa compared to heterosexual populations in other parts of the world and why the incidence of HIV infection in young women in southern Africa is so high".[80] This stunning confession of ignorance, made in 2012—three decades into the African HIV epidemics—indicates that the original question "Why Africa?" is still very much with us and, therefore, a crucial and urgent challenge. Any bets that comprehensive risk factor assessment, rather than the monochromatic focus on heterosexual sex, might help solve this puzzle?

Official negligence

In a thought-provoking essay, the German social scientist Moritz Hunsmann explored the political incentives of international health agencies and of African governments to dismiss or ignore evidence of non-sexual transmission in Africa's HIV epidemic.[81] In brief, he proposed that continued sexualization of the epidemic makes it easy to blame individual victims, whose personal behaviors (implied to be immoral) caused their disease. On the other hand, acknowledging an important role for non-sexual (puncturing) exposures in health, dental, cosmetic, and ritualistic settings would be politically threatening, because assuring healthcare and workplace safety would be viewed as the responsibility of governments and public health authorities. Implicit in his view is *official negligence*: deliberate underestimation, "if not outright denial", of non-sexual transmission, which exculpates governments and health agencies. To him, epidemiologists and researchers have been complicit, because they uncritically supported sexualization of Africa's HIV epidemics; furthermore, this turn of mind had a deleterious effect on rational evaluation of dissonances and anomalies ("conformist analysis inhibits reasonable debate") which "has done a lot of harm to both science and prevention policies".[81]

In a small series of papers[82–84] Gisselquist and colleagues[85] detailed errors of commission and omission by the public health establishment, donor agencies, and African governments. He states that public health authorities should be ashamed of themselves for the inadequate science and, therefore, missed prevention opportunities, not to mention the avoidable suffering[61] that resulted from both. What particularly irks him is what he views as the double standard, one for rich and one for poor countries, in HIV research ethics, epidemiologic science, and health care safety matters.[82] Double standards have enabled: 1) implementation of studies in which participants were not notified of their HIV-positive test, with all its implications for downstream transmission; 2) neglect for health care safety and for providing explicit warning about the dangers of unsanitary medical procedures; 3) failure to investigate unexplained infections by tracing and testing persons

215

exposed at about the same time in the same medical setting; 4) failure to conduct scientifically defensible studies to resolve dissonances; 5) and failure to publish empiric evidence suggestive of non-sexual transmission.[20,30,86] As he points out, such public health shortcomings would not have been tolerated in rich countries.

Emerging African voices

It remains remarkable that, three decades into the African HIV epidemics and more than a dozen years since our controversial papers suggested that the epidemiologic picture was not right, comprehensive investigations have still not been conducted by the international agencies responsible for effectively and confidently intervening in the sub-Saharan spread of HIV. One is unlikely to intervene effectively if the respective contributions of different modes of transmission are not solidly documented. In this regard, several groups of native investigators have recently voiced concern about the orthodox view stubbornly clung to by mainstream researchers.

First out of the gate in the new decade was Mapingure and his colleagues who published their puzzling findings in the *Journal of the International AIDS Society*. [87] The authors examined sexual risk factors for two groups of pregnant women, one from Zimbabwe and the other from Tanzania. Their aim was to elucidate risk factors that could explain the enormous difference in HIV prevalence: 26% in Zimbabwean, and 7% in Tanzanian, women. Counter-intuitively, risky sexual behaviors were more common among Tanzanian than Zimbabwean women. Differences in frequency of sexually transmitted infections among these women differed only moderately, while HIV infection differed by a factor of four. Intriguingly, a history of schistosomiasis was four times greater among Zimbabwean women, providing support for Sawers, Stillwaggon, and Hertz's view that such tropical diseases may influence HIV transmission, directly or indirectly.[74] Finally, the authors suggest that non-sexual routes of transmission might have played an important role in these substantial differences in HIV prevalence between the two countries, although such routes were regrettably not measured.

In an exceptionally well-done recent review of currently available information, Duri and Stray-Pedersen list observations that undermine the assertion that sexual transmission is mostly responsible for the observed high HIV prevalence in many regions of Africa.[88] They detail the multifarious dissonances, paradoxes, and shortcomings in the mainstream orthodox view and, importantly, offer suggestions for obtaining evidence on multiple fronts to solve this puzzle. Of particular concern to these two researchers, based at the University of Zimbabwe, is the real possibility that the pronounced differences noted in different regions of Africa could be explained by unsafe medical practices, such as the re-use of needles and other sharps. In any event, they recommend comprehensive study designs to examine the contributions of sexual behaviors, unsafe puncturing exposures, ethnic variation in HIV restriction genes, nutritional status in susceptible populations, viral characteristics, and co-infection with other pathogens that are common in Africa.

A 2014 article by a group of Kenyan researchers, analyzed data from the population-based representative national AIDS Indicator Survey to assess the magnitude of medical injection use and its relationship with HIV status. [89] In brief, the authors report that of nearly 14,000 participants, a little more than a third reported receiving one or more injections in the previous twelve months; of these, both men and women were about three times more likely to be HIV-positive than participants who did not report receiving injections during that interval. Unlike HIV researchers associated with international health agencies and principally European and North American universities, these African researchers may see things clearly not only because their friends and family are subject to the risks they consider, but also because they may not be subject to professional or financial pressures to conform to the consensus view. Perhaps, for them, questioning the orthodoxy would not be accompanied by threats of punishment or banishment. And yet, frankly, I am currently unconvinced that there will be sustained efforts on the part of skeptical Africans to solve the puzzle of rapid HIV transmission in their countries. Not only do I sense a certain passivity towards getting this thing done, but more disquieting is my guess that such a venture may not bring sufficient rewards. Dissenting or skeptical African researchers, it seems to me, are unlikely to be invited into international collaborations or granted funding. In my view, they would also be unlikely to be accorded status from their scientific peers, or accolades from their brethren who are working in government and in medicine. Indeed they could even earn their scorn. Am I misinterpreting the meager cues I've been exposed to in my work with AIDS in Africa, and thus being unduly pessimistic? I hope so.

As for non-African researchers the situation, based on this chapter's content, warrants pessimism. The depressing fact is that research on this topic ("Why Africa?") is dead. Here's this vibrant domain of research and controversy that I and my colleagues have been embroiled in for so many years and, with the exception of some offshoots and a few independent inquiries, as described above, all of the traditionally limited interest has seemingly fizzled.

"We do not believe any group of men adequate enough or wise enough to operate without scrutiny or without criticism. We know that the only way to avoid error is to detect it, that the only way to detect it is to be free to enquire. We know that the wages of secrecy are corruption. We know that in secrecy error, undetected, will flourish and subvert."

—Robert Oppenheimer

Twelve years before the mast: what I learned from this odyssey

Disappointment. Were I asked to confine myself to a single word to characterize the dozen or so years I spent thinking and writing about AIDS in Africa, this word gets the job done.

1. Disappointment with the failure of the international health agencies to commission scientifically rigorous studies after dissonances and anomalies were (relentlessly) pointed out.[90–93] A decade-and-a-half after these weaknesses in the official view were detailed, they continue to ignore or dismiss pertinent evidence. It is difficult to blame this failure on ignorance. For example, Dr. Peter Piot, director of the world's leading AIDS agency (UNAIDS) from its creation in 1995 until the end of 2008, was one of the earliest and savviest researchers on the ground in Africa with *Project SIDA* (French acronym for AIDS) in Kinshasa, Zaire. Here are the recommendations he published in the *African Journal of Sexually Transmitted Diseases* in 1986: "Other possible routes of transmission *that should be studied* include scarification rituals, tattooing, male and female circumcision and inadequate sterilization of needles re-used for medical treatment." And: "Further research is needed to accurately determine *all* risk factors for AIDS transmission in Africa, to determine the actual extent of AIDS, to work out control strategies, and determine the impact on other health facilities."[94] (Emphasis mine, in both sentences.) No one in our informal group could have articulated it better. Similar conclusions were published in the prestigious journal *Science* that same year.[95]

What happened? What made such researchers ignore their own considered, prescient advice? Or ours—and that of other skeptics—which was along similar lines? Finally, how many AIDS cases could have been prevented by conscientious implementation of these early researchers' advice? Or of other similarly minded researchers? 10,000? 100,000? 1,000,000? More? Finally, it does not engender trust in the official view to know that our informal group has solid evidence of several instances by international health agencies actively working to suppress findings supportive of non-sexual transmission and to discourage research into non-sexual transmission.[28,30,65,86,96]

2. Disappointment with the generally inadequate studies conducted by academic researchers from European, British, and North American universities. None implemented field studies that comprehensively took account of non-sexual exposures in sub-Saharan Africa or in other Third World countries. (If done, they were not published.) As Daniel Sarewitz pointed out: "A biased scientific result is no different from a useless one".[97] Their studies were almost always designed with "heterosexual transmission" as *the* frame of reference and, more often than not, relied on ecologic evidence,[31] anemic (read: missing non-sexual) risk factor assessment, inferential reasoning, and logic, rather than scientifically-relevant data. Worse, they were mired in group-think. What, to me, truly distorted epidemiological research was deference to unsound yet established theories of HIV transmission in Africa. (In fact this reminded me of the Western intelligentsia's misguided belief,

during the 1930s and 1940s, that Marxism/Utopian Communism would save humanity, and how this fervently-held belief blinded them to the brutalities of Soviet totalitarianism. True Believers saw what they wanted to see. Did AIDS academic researchers suffer from a similar intellectual straightjacket?)

3. Disappointment with the seemingly partisan leanings of scholarly journal editors, especially by editorial staff in high-impact journals. Not only did they generally reject our manuscripts, but they also often declined to publish our rebuttals to articles they published. This was our own, palpable introduction to publication bias.

"In the end, we will remember not the words of our enemies,
but the silence of our friends."
—Attributed to Martin Luther King, Jr.

4. Disappointment with so many (non-Colorado Springs) colleagues in the STD/HIV fields who remained silent on the sidelines, both officially and personally. Their reticence was difficult to understand not only because I had expected that, being scientifically trained, they would have greater respect for skepticism than for the received wisdom but, especially, because they knew of the high quality epidemiologic research I had done for decades. They certainly knew that I was—even if I personally lacked gravitas and had a reputation as a gadfly—an expert in STD/HIV epidemiology and control, having contributed

cutting-edge empiric studies for decades. And they knew that I certainly was not some sort of ideologue, whether Duesbergian or Mbekian denier, Anti-condomer, Anti-circumcisioner, or Pro-Abstinencer. True to my Swiss roots, I was neutral and pragmatic. I speculate that part of the reason for their silence may have been the same as it may have been for the international health agencies: the so-called Adverse Consequences Fallacy:[98] the error of evaluating the validity of an argument by considering its potential negative consequences. Whatever the cause of their silence, it was deafening and deeply disappointing.

5. Disappointment with the lack of truly scientific, as opposed to politically- or ideologically-motivated, debate. As I've said elsewhere: "I can only speculate about which comfort zones—ideological, political, programmatic, financial, academic—were threatened or could account for their failure to voice doubt, at least publicly. Was it due to inertia? To time-honored assumptions about African promiscuity? To not wanting to discourage Africans from seeking modern health care (e.g., immunizations, prenatal care)? To wishing it to be so? To hoping that condom use would enhance population control initiatives? To fears of losing comfortable funding streams? To constructing a sense of shared coping with Western homosexual men and injecting drug users? To fearing damage to academic or organizational reputation? To fears of public rebuke, scapegoating, or legal action? Painful as this process may turn out to be, answers to these questions must be sought."[33]

Two centuries ago, a German philosopher articulated this (probably relevant) insight: "How unwillingly we think of things which powerfully injure our interests, wound our pride, or interfere with our wishes, with what difficulty do we determine to lay such things before our intellects for careful and serious investigations…in that resistance of the will to allowing what is contrary to it to come under the examination of the intellect lies the place at which madness can break open the mind." (Schopenhauer, 1818)

6. Disappointment with misguided ad hominem comments. Other than the inappropriate name-calling referred to earlier, there were frequent and irritating instances of (irrelevant) deprecating comments. For example: "The American authors are not linked to a university."[99] (The authors referred to were Gisselquist and me.) The comment's intent was clearly to devalue our view, since it insinuates that valid work or critical thinking is not possible outside academia. I've often wondered how many readers of our papers dismissed their content based on similar considerations. Another not infrequently leveled accusation was that among our informal group were "scientists, some of whom have an insufficient understanding of basic epidemiological principles".[100] A truly gratuitous assessment, for it was unencumbered by evidence other than what the authors wanted to believe. Certainly the totality of our (the informal group) published work seriously challenged this belief. Along similar lines was the dismissive comment that our papers were: "…a propagandist message based on distinctly flimsy analysis and inference." This comment was emailed to the Royal Society of

Medicine on 19 April 2003 by a person who had been editor-in-chief of the prestigious *American Journal of Public Health*. It was certainly not lost on any of us that his assessment perfectly fit our view of the official version of HIV dynamics in Africa promulgated by the international health agencies! Many similar comments, made by people who should know better, were based on the arrogance of belief rather than the humility of doubt. Voltaire once said: "Doubt is not a very pleasant state, but certainty is a ridiculous one". This is a turn of mind regrettably missing from many in the international agencies and in academia who defend the consensus view.

Glimpsing into the future

It is entirely possible that we may never know what truly drove, and is currently driving, the HIV epidemics in sub-Saharan Africa. By dismissing or ignoring evidence that undermines the consensus view, mainstream agencies and researchers have effectively discouraged new research. The easiest way this is done is to refuse to fund proposals that challenge the consensus view or/and refuse to reward independent-minded researchers with advancement in academia.

No less a brilliant observer of enforced orthodoxy than George Orwell said it far better than I ever could:

> At any given moment there is an orthodoxy, a body of ideas of which it is assumed that all right-thinking people will accept without question. It is not exactly forbidden to say this, that or the other, but it is 'not done' to say it...Anyone who

challenges the prevailing orthodoxy finds himself silenced with surprising effectiveness. A genuinely unfashionable opinion is almost never given a fair hearing, either in the popular press or in high-brow periodicals.

Amen.

Again from Orwell:

The point is that we are all capable of believing things which we know to be untrue, and then, when we are finally proved wrong, impudently twisting the facts so as to show that we were right. Intellectually, it is possible to carry on this process for an indefinite time: the only check on it is that sooner or later a false belief bumps up against solid reality, usually on a battlefield.

The shocking recent report of hundreds of HIV infections in Roka village, western Cambodia, apparently due to skin puncturing medical procedures administered by a village practitioner may be such a battlefield.[101] This tragic outbreak can certainly serve as proof of concept that turbocharged HIV transmission can be generated by contaminated injections and other invasive medical procedures.

"Cultivate a taste for distasteful truths. And...
most important of all, endeavor to see things
as they are, not as they ought to be."
— Ambrose Pierce

The paradigm that failed: Phoenix should rise from its ashes

This was a difficult and, at times, painful chapter to write. And it is even more painful for an irrepressible optimist like me to end on a negative note. And so I won't.

We've come full circle and again ask: Why Africa? What is it about conditions in many parts of sub-Saharan Africa that HIV is so efficiently transmitted in its heterosexual populations, a phenomenon experienced nowhere else on earth? The short answer still is: we don't *know*. I certainly don't know. But neither do they—"they" being the international health agencies and the preponderance of the academic researchers who study HIV transmission in Africa. And certainly, shortcomings in our arguments do not, ipso facto, provide support for the consensus view. The quality of the evidence they rely on for asserting that unprotected penile-vaginal intercourse accounts for the vast majority of infections in African adults is not high enough to be scientifically trustworthy. Were their assertion not undermined by persistent evidence suggesting a substantial role for non-sexual HIV transmission, there would be little reason to worry about quality of evidence. Indeed, it is the multifarious facts that don't fit which demand a higher standard of evidence. Neither weak evidence nor wishful thinking can get the job done of persuading thinking people that the present consensus view is correct. It is especially disconcerting to note that, with so much at stake for implementing correctly targeted interventions in Africa, there has been such stubborn and sustained reluctance on the part of researchers and international health agencies to resolve incongruities and get the picture right, using comprehensive research designs. It is even more disconcerting to realize that they had twice recommended[32] or promised[26] to look into non-sexual modes of transmission and twice failed to follow through.

What does one say about a paradigm, promulgated as the consensus view more than a quarter of a century ago, that has not been modified since, in light of respectable evidence, old and new, clearly indicating the need to revisit this view? The answer can only be: ossified dogma— dogma maintained by the weight of authority and tradition, not quality evidence. And one can only speculate, as I did above, about the vested interests maintaining what Dr. Gisselquist calls the epiganda (a contraction of "epidemiologic propaganda") which discourages taking a fresh look. At the very least, readers should ask the establishment researchers and health agencies charged with monitoring and intervening in HIV epidemics why they have settled for evidence from a lesser god when the stakes for getting the picture right are so high.[35] Africans need a picture based on rigorous epidemiologic science. What they have received so far, regrettably, is more political, than rigorous, science. Africans deserve better than the inadequately supported views of the heterosexual transmission fundamentalists.

There is a way forward. Its starting point is to recruit the best possible epidemiologic study designs and conscientiously implement them in several different regions of sub-Saharan Africa. Above all there is ample reason to care, on the deepest level, because taking a fresh look is far more about humanitarian considerations than about rigorous science.

EPILOGUE

"Nothing great was ever achieved without enthusiasm"
—Ralph Waldo Emerson

We loved our work. That was its most transparent characteristic—evident to our patients, clients, co-workers, colleagues, the local media, and the larger community. Without it, few of the successes detailed in this book would have been achieved; it was without question the key ingredient.

Another crucial ingredient was luck. (Asked what qualities he sought in his commanders, Napoleon replied: "Give me lucky generals". He did not trust skill, training, or brains as much as luck.) And how lucky we were. Let me count the ways.

The seven pillars of success

Geography: we worked in an area that was discretely bounded, 40 to 65 miles distant from other population centers in any direction. This made it relatively easy to validly measure the impact of our STD/HIV interventions, since they were not directly influenced by those implemented in neighboring public health jurisdictions.

Bureaucratic structure: our local health department was largely independent of the State health department in Denver (65 miles away) which, in any event, granted much local autonomy for responding to local problems. There was no heavy, arrogant, top-down administrative pressure. Collegiality ruled.

Leadership: The director of our local health department traditionally supported and facilitated STD control. This support flowered under the exceptional leadership of John B. Muth, MD who was our health department director for nearly two decades starting in 1980. Incisive intelligence, wisdom, integrity, courage, political savvy, and tolerance for dissent made for an ideal management style. Failure to thrive programmatically under these leadership conditions was virtually impossible.

Employee loyalty: Most employees signed up (as it were) for the duration, despite the lack of vertical mobility and generally low salaries. Long-term employees were the rule during the last three decades of the 20th century. These seasoned veterans of the STD/HIV programs were principally motivated by the challenges of this difficult craft and, above all, by the intrinsic rewards of altruism. They were making a palpable difference and they knew it. In brief: the work was its own reward.

Lack of "prima donna" staff members: physicians in our STD/HIV clinics not only were comfortable with our patients and their occasionally exotic behaviors, but they were humble: simple humility in some, genuine tolerance and curiosity in others.

Being there at the right time: in the early days physicians, who were trained in the individual patient professional paradigm, were usually in charge of STD programs and budget priorities in the United States. Hence, little empiric research had been done on the *community*, as opposed to *clinical*, form of STD. This reality presented an opportunity to investigate the community form of STD in a largely unchartered (and prima facie unglamorous) field.

First-rate collaborators: it is astonishing that a minor STD/HIV program in a minor health jurisdiction near the middle of the United States (read: away from the influential public health centers usually located on the coasts) was able to attract and retain the services of first-rate conceptual and analytic minds to help discipline its empiric investigations. It is even more astonishing that their services were modestly compensated or, more often, freely given.

The road taken

With infections that are spread person-to-person by direct contact, it is the most natural thing in the world to do contact tracing. One goes upstream to find out where infection originated and downstream to find out where it might have propagated. Conceptually easy, it is difficult to do. Persuading STD patients to reveal the most intimate secrets of their lives—with whom they have sex, where, in what ways, how often—takes self-confidence, imagination and, above all, tenacity. It takes a special kind of person to volunteer in the first place, and an especially motivated one to stick with the craft for more than a few months. Turnover in contact tracing personnel is customarily high.

As luck would have it, I was able to attract, fund, and retain high quality contact tracers, most of whom stayed with me for many years. Part of this longevity is attributable to my assigning tasks that played to their strengths—without being overly concerned about their weaknesses since, in our team, one person's weakness was often compensated by another person's strength—and part is attributable to my frequent reminders that their work was valuable and valued. Not a year went by without my providing detailed summaries of contact tracing outcomes and interpreting their impact (the "valuable" part), not to mention conveying my personal appreciation, as well as our administration's and community's (the "valued" part). And talk about phenomenal output: between 1972 and 2000, a period during which a total of about 55,000 cases of reportable STD (gonorrhea, chlamydia, syphilis, and HIV/AIDS) were recorded, two-thirds were successfully interviewed for sexual partner information, naming an average of 1.7 partners per interview. Little wonder that our STD/HIV programs received numerous local, state, and national awards during these decades (See Appendix 3); note that most of the key contact tracers received individual awards.

As director of the STD/HIV department I was keenly aware of my responsibility to the public; it was their tax money that funded our programs and clinics. Not only did I feel that I owed them our best possible efforts but I insisted on documenting our performance with solid data. We were, first and last, a numerate program—"Show me the numbers" was my motto. This was the original impulse behind the meticulous documentation of our activities. It was only later that I realized (was made to realize?) that our quality data, continuously collected over many years, could be used to contribute to the epidemiologic literature. Most of our publications were a byproduct of doing our job really well—with enthusiasm and pride. Enthusiasm came effortlessly—I've been accused of being "unreasonably happy"— and it seemingly "infected" those around me.

As for my interest in writing well and in science/mathematics, an academic streak seems to run in my family. An uncle, Jean-Charles Potterat, was a *Belle Lettrist* trained at the Sorbonne, specializing in poetry; his son Olivier has a PhD in phytology and is a researcher in pharmacology in Basel (naturally); my nephew Eric Potterat, with a PhD in psychology, does stress and survival skills research with the U.S. Navy's SEALS in San Diego. My own two children, one a health care administrator for the indigent and the other, a math/science teacher, share their parents' love of learning and are widely-read. Maybe apples don't fall far from trees. But maybe they do, for my father was a fine-pastry and -candy confectioner.

"I do not greatly care whether I have been right or wrong on any point, but I care a good deal about which of the two I have been."

—Samuel Butler

Conclusion

The take-home message is that one can accomplish a lot with low-tech interventions like conscientious contact tracing—once called the sleeping giant of sexually transmissible disease control—unglamorous as it might be. Not only did this activity—our core programmatic function, the Swiss Army knife of epidemiology—impact the STD/HIV burdens in our own community (control), but it yielded insights into transmission dynamics (epidemiology) that formed the basis for our evidence-based control initiatives. Contact tracing not only had a positive impact on our local disease burdens, but it illuminated aspects of transmission dynamics that have received international recognition. Most of this recognition sprang from the nearly 200 publications that appeared in the medical and public health literature. These articles have garnered more than 3,300 citations in the (conservative) *International Scientific Index* and more than 6,200 in (the more inclusive) *Google Scholar*, thanks to a little help from numerous friends and colleagues. At last count (Spring 2015), for example, there were 145 different co-authors featured on these 200 publications, in which I am first author on nearly half (and on 80% as first or second author).

To know that we have given contact tracing—a discipline that has been disrespected and underused since the arrival of AIDS in the early 1980s—and its academic twin, network analysis, solid empiric support, and to know that we have often broken new ground in our investigations by exploring their many offerings, fills us with the satisfaction of a professional life well-lived. It was a good thing to have done. Currently, contact tracing continues to be used, most commonly to investigate infectious disease outbreaks, such as TB, measles, polio, emerging respiratory syndromes, or periodically re-emerging infections like Ebola—and regrettably less commonly with classic sexually transmissible and blood-borne infections.[1]

Parting shot

This book may well provide a sense, if not a measure, for what was lost as a consequence of public health authorities permitting contact tracing to fall into disuse in the United States.

Sleeping giant: awake!

APPENDIX ONE

INFORMATION SYSTEMS

(Edited for content accuracy by Stephen Q. Muth)

The notable STD control achievements detailed in this book occurred in a period when substantial improvements in data storage and information technology were being made in the United States. At the core of these improvements during the last thirty years of the 20th century was the electronic computer—initially the mainframe, then the mini, followed by the personal, computer.

Until the mid-1980s, all our documents were maintained in paper files, because the STD program did not yet own a computer. (Indeed we were lucky to own a single IBM Selectric[1] typewriter, bought in the mid-1970s!) The game changer was HIV counseling and testing, a national initiative funded through the CDC in mid-1985, which provided the means for local programs to afford personal computers (PCs). Prior to the arrival of PCs in our STD/HIV section, access to computers meant occasional use of mainframes[2] or minis[3] at the State Health Department, at the CDC, or at the local branch of the

---

[1] IBM "Selectric I/O Keyboard Printer" manual: http://media.ibm1130.org/E0033.pdf

[2] IBM "360 Model 30" mainframe (picture)
http://www-03.ibm.com/ibm/history/exhibits/mainframe/mainframe_2423PH2030.html

[3] https://en.wikipedia.org/wiki/VAX_8000#VAX_8600

University of Colorado. These computers were used to enter and analyze data stemming exclusively from our special epidemiologic studies. The only routine program data entered and stored on any computer were results from specimens we shipped—as we did all HIV and hepatitis tests—to the State reference laboratory in Denver, starting in mid-1985.

Enter Stephen Q. Muth, Whiz Kid of Information Technology (IT)

If the national HIV/AIDS counseling and testing initiative provided sufficient funding for us to gradually begin using computers in support of routine STD program tasks, then it was our network epidemiology initiative in the late 1980s (Project 90: See Chapter 6) that revolutionized our STD/HIV programs' data storage and analytic capabilities. And the chief architect for these computer programming achievements was Steve Muth, a young college graduate in biochemistry with a brilliant, probing mind, and a talent for making computers do his bidding. His fierce intelligence was matched by his tenacity and stamina. For Steve, all IT problems admitted of solutions, even if he had to take thorny challenges home and do all-nighters until the problem was solved. Although originally hired under the auspices of Project 90 in 1988 as the project's data manager, he gradually developed information systems that would, in time, form a comprehensive infrastructure unifying both STD and HIV programs' clinic and outreach activities. From the modest beginnings of simply counting disease cases, to pegging them in social and geographic space, to modeling contact tracing networks, through developing a user-friendly system to integrate these functions beneath a centralized patient registry, the technology originally developed for Project 90 would ultimately assist all data functions from simple chart management to longitudinal geospatial network analysis.

The state of the art in 1988

It is worth remembering that, while small computers had been around for more than 10 years by 1988, for most people they were little more than glorified typewriters. (Even the Centers for Disease Control had yet to devise computer-based record keeping for local STD/HIV surveillance and contact tracing personnel to use—the future STD*MIS[4] system, released in 1991. Steve's first task was to use dedicated database software to solve data management issues, using the STD Program's brand new $3,000 33-MHz 386 IBM clone.[5] An important constraint was tight department budgeting that forced our health department to forgo relatively expensive office software, like Lotus 1-2-3,[6] for less expensive alternatives, like Ashton-Tate's Framework.[7] Framework was supposed to be in a similar class as Lotus, promising to put word processing, spreadsheets, and databases under one roof. A key problem was available personal computer memory;

---

[4] https://health.state.tn.us/STD/PDFs/STDMIS_User_Manual.pdf

[5] http://en.wikipedia.org/wiki/IBM_Personal_Computer/AT#Clones

[6] https://en.wikipedia.org/wiki/Lotus_1-2-3

[7] https://en.wikipedia.org/wiki/Framework_(office_suite)

special drivers and hardware setups were necessary to make use of "upper" and "extended" memory (the region above 640k), and use of such memory was an absolute requirement for growing databases. The STD/HIV Program had the most expensive computer in the building, with an expanded memory card,[8] and a 30 megabyte removable Tandon hard drive[9] which could be locked away in the health department's central vault at night, but once the HIV-testing database grew past 3,000 records, swapping between memory and glacially slow hard drives became a bottleneck, causing each search for the numeric patient charts to take five to ten minutes. The Framework solution, which had worked fine for a few years, eventually precipitated a crisis.

As luck would have it, Jerry Macon, a local entrepreneur, had acquired Stoneware Systems' Advanced DB Master (ADBM)[10] line of database software for the Apple II, and had recompiled it to work under MS-DOS, our computer platform. His team was also hard at work, making it compatible with "expanded", then "extended" memory. ADBM was at that time a "flat-file" database, capable of holding only one table in memory at a time. ("Relational" databases—like Oracle[11] and dBase[12]— existed then and could relate multiple tables to each other, but like

---

[8] https://en.wikipedia.org/wiki/Expanded_memory

[9] http://www.ccapitalia.net/galeria/main.php?g2_itemId=329

& http://nrdblog.cmosnet.eu/2011/10/zegnaj-nrd-update-tandon-pac-286/#axzz3pHKitGij

[10] http://www.maconsys.com/AboutADBM.aspx

[11] http://docs.oracle.com/cd/B19306_01/server.102/b14220/intro.htm

[12] https://en.wikipedia.org/wiki/DBase

most good things, were priced out of our reach, and tended to require computer experts for support.) [13] ADBM was relatively simple, affordably priced for small businesses, and had a manageable learning curve.

A detail that would prove to be a critical asset, ADBM required that the database user assign "unique primary keys"[14] as the first fields in every record. Other, more sophisticated database packages had no such restriction, allowing developers more freedom to design their own (sometimes illogical) record configurations. ADBM's design was perfect for a person without specific training in information systems management—and very little spare time—who needed to design lightning-fast systems that were logically consistent. It forced one to organize records into systems indexed by fields whose combinations were unique.

Initially, an ADBM database was a so-called "flat file"[15], meaning data tables were not interlinked. The HIV-testing-record flat file (ATSDBASE, see Chapter 3) was the first database to be created, to solve the immediate problem of accessing records in a numeric (because clients being tested for HIV feared to be listed by name) filing

---

[13] In the El Paso County Health Department of the late 80s, Steve and John Muth were the sole persons able to act as software specialists and computer maintenance technicians; they provided *de facto* support for the entire health department's needs.

[14] https://en.wikipedia.org/wiki/Unique_key

[15] https://en.wikipedia.org/wiki/Flat_file_database

system. Next, LADYJANE (See Chapter 5) was created to catalog visits to our clinic by prostitute women. This, then, was the rather anemic computing environment at the time: a single 386DX machine, the backbone of the office and one portable Toshiba 286.

As described in Chapter 6, Dr. Klovdahl arrived from Australia to help design Project 90 survey instruments and, crucially, to design its databases. Again financial considerations constrained the solutions. Dr. Klovdahl wanted to work with SAS (Statistical Analysis System); we had bought the cheaper Systat. He wanted dBase; we had the cheaper ADBM. Despite the completely fish-out-of-water situation he was thrust into, he designed an admirable database for Project 90 within the constraints of flat files. The example that Dr. Klovdahl set for us in that one system of data tables would provide the template for all of our subsequent clinic and program databases.

In a very short order, Steve decided to give our 386DX computer an expanded memory board (4 Megs), plus a fancy newly-invented kind of hard drive (a miraculous 160 Megs of storage!). In addition, Steve had to stay current with the latest utilities needed to compress and encrypt our sensitive data. Most importantly, we capitulated to Dr. Klovdahl's (expensive) suggestion that we obtain, at least, Base SAS. This analysis program would turn out to be the #1 tool in both academic and upper-level government environments; had the best software engineers in the world working to improve it, and consequently had the most fine-tuned control of any high-level programming language [16] then in existence. It was a perfect backdrop with which Steve could exercise various techniques he had already learned prior to joining our organization. Steve's academic training in chemical engineering as an undergraduate at the University of Colorado, Boulder during the early 1980s emphasized computing and logic circuits. Thus, not only had he been exposed to computer languages (e.g., Pascal, Fortran, Basic, and even 6502 machine code), but also to programs for inverting matrices and for finding eigenvectors—keys for unraveling network analysis programs such as GRADAP[17] and UCINet 3.0,[18] acquired shortly after attending his first network conference in 1990.[19] In a remarkably short time, Steve was developing SAS programs to solve our principal challenge—data quantity (over 8,000 nodes) that exceeded the limitations (6,000 nodes and 60,000 dyads) of GRADAP, the best DOS PC-based network analysis software then available.

So despite the fact that Steve was not a computer scientist versed in the most advanced techniques of the day, he was using software designed by people who were. Moreover, he had just enough old-school

---

[16] https://en.wikipedia.org/wiki/High-level_programming_language

[17] **GRA**ph **D**efinition and **A**nalysis **P**ackage. Release 2.10, 10 February 1992. No longer available from iec PROGAMMA, Gröningen, The Netherlands. The original version dates back to January 1982. http://link.springer.com/article/10.3758%2FBF03202113

[18] MacEvoy B and Freeman L. UCINET 3.0, Irvine CA. Mathematical Social Science Group, School of Social Sciences, University of California, 1987. Later: Borgatti S, Everett M and Freeman L. UCINET IV Version 1.0. Columbia: Analytic Technologies, 1992. Latest version currently available from Steve Borgatti at his website: http://www.analytictech.com

[19] X[th] International Social Networks "Sunbelt" Conference, San Diego, CA, February 1990.

programming techniques learned as a teenager (e.g. simple binary searches,[20] use of elementary pointers,[21] vectors[22] and arrays[23] for simple direct access[24]), which when combined with his stubborn persistence, served to knit various software packages together to make integrated systems that were usually greater than the sum of their parts. For example, instead of approaching each analytical procedure as a one-time task to find an answer and to then move on to the next challenge, Steve was in constant search of general ways to automate virtually everything that was done, so that end-users in our department had keystroke macros[25] to bring very complicated types of record searches and data analyses within reach of the rest of the STD/HIV team of computer neophytes. Automating record searches was to have far-reaching consequences later.

The end of Project 90

By 1992, when data collection for Project 90 officially concluded, we thus had both office and program personnel with the ability to instantaneously locate relevant records: HIV testing charts, Project 90 respondents and their contacts, prostitute women, as well as key

---

[20] https://en.wikipedia.org/wiki/Binary_search_algorithm#Iterative

[21] https://en.wikipedia.org/wiki/Pointer_(computer_programming)

[22] https://en.wikipedia.org/wiki/Array_data_structure#One-dimensional_arrays

[23] https://en.wikipedia.org/wiki/Array_data_structure#Multidimensional_arrays

[24] https://en.wikipedia.org/wiki/Random_access

[25] https://en.wikipedia.org/wiki/Macro_(computer_science)#Keyboard_and_mouse_macros

people associated with the transmission of STD, especially gonorrhea. Finally granted, after 4 years as a Project 90 data manager, a full-time position as an Information Systems Manager, Steve took this opportunity to conceptualize and implement an inexpensive network to serve all of our programs in the STD/HIV department. Above all, he made sure this computer information-hub was not connected to the main health department computer network, and would remain so because of cable-length constraints.

This independence allowed Steve to do things that are now probably no longer possible in a local county government bureaucracy. He combed want ads and local garage sales to find bargains on obsolete computers and accessories. There was no IT department to override his decisions and no purchasing officer to go through. I simply trusted him to order only what was needed, and to obtain the equipment at bargain basement prices. In this way, Steve built a network, starting with the contact tracers each having a "dumb terminal" (now called "thin clients"[26]) that could access the rapidly expanding databases served by a central 486 machine (the "super tower").

The Project 90 social and geographic analysis period

By 1994, Project 90 analysis requirements once again helped direct the development of our STD/HIV programs' IT infrastructure. As

---

[26] https://en.wikipedia.org/wiki/Thin_client

described in Chapter 6, we had requested additional funding to do advanced analyses using Project 90 data, especially to investigate network dynamics in geographic space (via geocoding[27] and spatial analyses[28]). Luckily, by now, our county government had benefitted from federal grants to support its own geographical information systems (GIS) department, with teams of people sent into the field to digitally map our streets, blocks, block groups and census tracts. Consequently, we upgraded our DOS-based mapping software, Atlas Graphics, using its successor in the Windows world, which would become Arcview by ESRI. [29] Arcview, it turns out by fortunate coincidence, was a subset of the same package our county government was using to map our area with unprecedented precision, which is exactly what we were able to do with our contact tracing and risk networks data.

The later 1990s: Steve Muth's search for the
STD/HIV computerized data Holy Grail

Steve's view of the Holy Grail of STD/HIV data systems was a work environment in which real-time—as opposed to retrospective—data analysis/feedback would guide contact tracers in their quotidian tasks and interventions. Instead of being weeks to months behind the epidemiologic events (actual STD/HIV transmission), as had been

---

[27] https://en.wikipedia.org/wiki/Geocoding

[28] https://en.wikipedia.org/wiki/Spatial_analysis

[29] https://en.wikipedia.org/wiki/ArcView_3.x

done since time immemorial, Steve armed each contact tracer with an (affordable) secondhand computer. Since top priority was generally the newest information coming from the clinic or from field investigations, the central IT challenge was how to quickly clean-up and collate these incoming data. This not only facilitated the task of closing the required paperwork but, more crucially, it allowed contact tracers to rapidly assess any named contact's position in their transmission network: central, hence high priority, or peripheral, hence low(er) priority.

While the impetus to function in real time was Steve's ambitious dream, the modus operandi was inspired by Project 90, because the problem faced in Project 90 was similar: we needed to identify partners named in STD/HIV contact interviews—whose identifying information was frequently marginal—with as much precision as possible. For years we had manually analyzed lists of persons named by others as sexual or drug partners; we needed to hunt through these lists looking for matches to prevent duplication of actors in risk networks. We now needed to keep all STD/HIV programs', not just Project 90, databases as free of duplicates as possible. The central challenge was to develop reliable matching algorithms when sifting through imperfect data such as missing or misspelled names, partial addresses or locating information, phone numbers, aliases, name variants, different people with similar names living together, name changes due to change in civil status, sloppy handwriting, not to mention data entry error. Readers interested in greater detail are referred to our Oxford University Press chapter. [30] Steve devised, entirely in his spare time, trustworthy algorithms. Steve did not know it at the time, but he was independently inventing what is now called "fuzzy matching" software. [31] (Similar fuzzy matching software has since been designed independently to de-duplicate the National Cancer Registry, and is now freely available as RegistryPlus™ LinkPlus [32]). Nothing even remotely resembling this software was available then and, modesty aside, Steve's homespun software to this day (2015) remains superior in some respects: how it handles name variants, phonetic variants, and weightings of importance of various match elements.

Although the challenges inherent in permuting records based on multiple aliases had been solved (for generating Project 90 name listings by 1989), the rise of the World Wide Web in the late 90s opened a new world of opportunities. One such opportunity, discovered in late 1997 when Steve started using the new search engine GOOGLE, presented itself in the form of an exhaustive list of name variants maintained by a Tennessee genealogist interested in cataloging baby names, Judy Henley Phillips. After obtaining her permission—it turned out she was delighted to contribute to the disease control enterprise—Steve now received an exhaustive dataset of Anglo-Saxon

---

[30] Potterat JJ, Woodhouse DE, Muth SQ, Rothenberg RB, Darrow WW, Klovdahl AS, Muth JB. Network dynamism: history and lessons of the Colorado Springs study, in Morris M (ed.). *Network Epidemiology: A Handbook for Survey Design and Data Collection.* Oxford University Press Inc., New York 2004: 87–114. http://www.oup.co.uk/isbn/0-19-926901-7

[31] https://en.wikipedia.org/wiki/Record_linkage#Probabilistic_record_linkage

[32] http://www.cdc.gov/cancer/npcr/tools/registryplus/lp_features.htm

/ Hispanic / Germanic name equivalents (e.g., William / Wilhelm / Bill, or Jack / John, or Jeff / Geoffrey).[33] Using computer expertise no more advanced than SAS, binary searches, use of pointers and arrays to directly access records, and a penchant for optimizing code, Steve was able to create an algorithm which substantially reduced the number of potential match candidates (a process now known as "blocking" or in this case, making multiple blocking passes). In addition to this multiple-name problem, Steve's new algorithm improved the sifting process by using phonetic equivalents and via another simple technique for matching strings based on adjacent two- and three-letter sequences which reduced problems caused by errant spellings, data entry error, and sloppy handwriting. Most of these solutions (name variants, fuzzy matching of strings) became readily available because of the web, and others (like blocking and phonetic conversion) Steve ended up inventing independently, unaware of advances that had been made in the computing field in the 1980s.

In another fortuitous turn of events, in 1997 Slovenia, the team of Andrej Mrvar and Vladimir Batagelj produced freeware (our price range!) called "Pajek"[34] for visualizing large networks. Their program could read ASCII text files for input (simple enough for computer-unsophisticated people to understand). Steve was now poised to implement two crucial operational innovations: real-time network

---

[33] http://www.tngenweb.org/franklin/frannick.htm

[34] http://vlado.fmf.uni-lj.si/pub/networks/pajek/

analysis in socio-geographic space, and the integration of all our disparate STD/HIV/Hepatitis databases under a single system.

2001—The Killing Fields of bureaucracy

Steve and I retired (early 2001), but Steve kept his word by working with County IT for the next six months, bringing a real-time STD/HIV/Hepatitis IT system to fruition. But despite seven subsequent years where remaining members of the STD/HIV team demonstrated the system's ease of use and utility, the health department's higher authorities terminated their collaboration with the County Information Services Department, dismantling what was probably the most comprehensive database system for STI/HIV/Hepatitis surveillance and control in existence. In addition, by the end of 2008, the STD/HIV Programs were permanently dissolved; not even a skeleton crew remained.

The End.

APPENDIX TWO

FORMAL ENGAGEMENT: OUR LETTERS TO THE EDITOR

Although busy on the front lines of STD/HIV control, where daily duties were as demanding and relentless as those for parenting young children, I considered it important not only to try to keep up with the relevant published literature, but to also actively participate, when qualified, in commenting on its content.

And so it was that, for more than a quarter century I was directly involved in writing 107 scholarly letters to the editor, 70% of which were published. As detailed in the annotated bibliography below, between 1986 and 2013, 75 letters appeared in the (principally) refereed literature and 32 were not published.

Given the fierce competition for inclusion in the modest amount of space allocated to letters in journals, this is a striking record, both quantitatively and qualitatively. That these published letters were essentially authored by a correspondent without advanced academic qualifications—nearly ninety percent of published letters feature me as first or second author—many of which originated from a control program practicing STD/HIV control in a minor leagues health department is notable. In addition, this exceptional output testifies to our deep commitment to advancing the field, and not just the activities, of STD/HIV control.

Publication is just that: it makes thinking public. Debate via letters to the editor not only forces one to put one's thinking cap on, but clearly exposes strengths and (alas) shortcomings in one's views, a process which is essential in epidemiologic science. Nothing intellectually ventured, nothing gained. Here, then, are our contributions to this process, some of which are annotated to give the reader a sense for the issues:

I. Published Letters to the Editor that I Authored or Co-authored

1. Potterat JJ, Muth JB, Markewich GS.   Serological markers as indicators of sexual orientation in AIDS-virus infected men. *Journal of the American Medical Association* 1986; 256: 712.

   Offers actuarial technique to validate self-reports of risk factors by men with HIV using specific blood tests ("Patients may lie, but blood doesn't" idea).

2. Potterat JJ, Phillips L, Muth JB. Lying to military physicians about risk factors for HIV infections. *Journal of the American Medical Association* 1987; 257: 1727.

   Provocative study that undermined the assertion by Walter Reed doctors that military men with HIV acquired it differently (heterosexually, from prostitutes) than their civilian counterparts (homosexually or via injecting drug use). Our interviews demonstrated that soldiers' risk factors mirrored those in the civilian sector and that they had lied to military doctors (because their doctors worked for the soldiers' employers). Incendiary title provided by JAMA editors, not us!

3. Potterat JJ. Does syphilis facilitate acquisition of HIV? *Journal of the American Medical Association* 1987; 258: 473–474.

   First empiric evidence that syphilis infection (via lesions) might facilitate sexual transmission of HIV. Early suggestion that syphilis patients should routinely be offered HIV testing and that blacks should be informed, as a high priority, of their very high risk for HIV infection.

4. Potterat JJ. "B" stands for bursa or its equivalent, bone. *Journal of the American Medical Association* 1988; 259: 1811.

   Short query about the origin of nomenclature for our immune system's B-cells.

5. Potterat JJ, Muth JB, Woodhouse DE. Discussing the implications of HIV infection in health care workers. *Journal of Acquired Immune Deficiency Syndromes* 1989; 2: 308–309.

Makes estimates of the number and proportion of HIV-infected health care workers in the United States and reminds them that transmission can be bi-directional (from infected health care worker to patient). Suggests convening expert panel to explore implications.

6. Potterat JJ, Muth JB, Murray C. Partner notification. *Annals of Internal Medicine* 1990; 113: 481.

    Disagrees with editorial which concludes that STD partner notification (contact tracing) is not efficacious. Explains that its author fails to see the forest for the trees: contact tracing appears ineffectual at the individual tree (case interview) level and may be most efficacious at the forest (core group) level.

7. Potterat JJ. HIV infection in rural Florida women. *New England Journal of Medicine* 1993; 328: 1351–1352.

    Criticizes CDC study claiming that women in rural Florida were infected through heterosexual transmission when, in fact, the authors failed to collect data on anal intercourse. (The authors reply that high-risk women in Florida do indeed practice anal sex.)

8. Muth JB, Potterat JJ. Condom courage. *The Medical Reporter* 1994; 2 (10): 4.

    Argues that medical knowledge is a trust and that doctors have a duty to offer accurate harm-reduction information to patients, free of ideological or religious constraints.

9. Potterat JJ, Rothenberg RB. Acquired immunity to gonorrhea? *Sexually Transmitted Diseases* 1995; 22: 261–264.

    Uses reasoning and data to undermine Brunham and colleagues' conclusion that infection with gonorrhea and chlamydia confers immunity, especially in populations that are repeatedly exposed.

10. Potterat JJ, Muth JB. Core groups by any other name? *Sexually Transmitted Diseases* 1996; 23: 164–165.

    Opposes CDC-proposed nomenclature change from "core groups" to "spread clusters", arguing that name change must reflect what has been learned since core groups were christened. Proposes "core networks" as being more concordant with current understanding of transmission dynamics: the shift from focus on core populations (people) to network conformation (structure).

11. Plummer L, Potterat JJ, Muth SQ, Muth JB, Darrow WW. Providing support and assistance for low-income or homeless women. *Journal of the American Medical Association* 1996; 276: 1874–1875.

    Response to a JAMA article advocating that women in economic and social crises be assisted to assure access to ameliorative social services, via professional case management. Presented are data on 67 women at high–risk for crises (young prostitutes and their closely matched controls) who were offered such services in a rigorously supportive manner. Efforts were labor intensive and modestly successful and failed to assure that the women would avail themselves of needed services, probably because of mental disorders (e.g., clinical depression, post-traumatic stress…)

12. Potterat JJ, Rothenberg RB. Sexual network data help assess putative STD reporting bias. *Sexually Transmitted Diseases* 1997; 24: 552–553.

Provides empiric network data to show that frequent sexual mixing between black men and white women in gonorrhea transmission accounts for the under-representation of white men in case reports (viz., it's not an artifact of private physicians under-reporting cases in white men).

13. Potterat JJ. Flawed syphilis analysis. *Science News* 1999; 155: 51.

Criticizes the CDC conclusion that the late-1990s Baltimore syphilis outbreak was caused by crack-cocaine prostitution and decrements in public health services. Associates outbreak with the contemporaneous implosion of public housing, which shattered social networks and dispersed syphilis transmitters to other parts of Baltimore (syphilis diaspora, as it were).

14. Potterat JJ, Muth SQ. Of vice and men: reflections on drug abuse and male prostitution. *Sexually Transmitted Diseases* 1999; 26: 93–94.

Questions article that sees prostitution by male injecting drug users as economically motivated; infers that it's more likely to be a function of characterological and/or psychological factors.

15. Potterat JJ, Brody S. Interpretation of research on sexual abuse of boys. *Journal of the American Medical Association* 1999; 281:2185–2186.

Critiques JAMA review of childhood sexual abuse, pointing out that researcher bias (evidenced by frequent use of "sequelae") and retrospective study design contribute to confusing association with causation. Calls for consideration of "upstream" variables, such as preexisting psychological susceptibility or disorders in respondents, before concluding how much of downstream morbidity is related to childhood sexual abuse.

16. Brody S, Potterat JJ. RE: "Is there really a heterosexual AIDS epidemic in the United States? Findings from a multisite validation study: 1992–1995". *American Journal of Epidemiology* 1999; 150: 429–430.

Criticizes as inadequate the CDC decision rules for assigning AIDS cases to the "heterosexual" category. Recommends use of multi-method searches of invalidating patients' self-reports of risk factors and use of specific biological markers. Also recommends replacing the ambiguous and confounded CDC classificatory system for AIDS/HIV to more precisely reflect specific high-risk behaviors (e.g., receptive anal intercourse).

17. Potterat JJ, Brody S. More of the same is not validation. *Sexually Transmitted Diseases* 2000; 27: 60–61.

Criticizes article that views use of multiple sources of patient self-reports as validation; such an approach gauges reliability, not validity. Advocates use of quality clinical and laboratory evidence for markers of high-risk behaviors (e.g., hepatitis-C testing). Regrettably, health workers probing for risk factors place more emphasis on civility (fear of offending) than on scientific accuracy.

18. Brewer D, Potterat JJ. Named-based surveillance for HIV-infected persons. *Annals of Internal Medicine* 2000; 132; 922–923.

Criticizes a study of HIV patients, who reportedly notified their own partners, for failing to validate these claims. Presents empiric evidence undermining their unvalidated assertion.

19. Potterat JJ, Muth SQ, Brody S.   Evidence undermining the adequacy of the HIV reproductive number formula. *Sexually Transmitted Diseases* 2000; 27: 644–645.

   Theoretic and empiric evidence are presented undermining the adequacy of the STD/HIV field's most central mathematical formula: R=B c (x) D. The crucial parameter "c" fails to take network structure (spatial conformation of contact patterns) into account. Usefulness may depend on scale.

20. Potterat JJ, Dowe T, Brewer DD.   Response to Who among us? (Review). *Journal of Sex Research* 2000; 37: 387–388.

   Response to book review stating that Colorado Springs had the highest concentration of prostitutes in the United States and that much of it was connected to cadets at the Air Force Academy. Data are presented to rebuke author's view, which was unencumbered by real data.

21. Potterat JJ, Muth SQ, Stites HK.   Twenty-year mortality in a 1981 cohort of homosexuals with gonorrhoea: a preliminary estimate. *International Journal of STD & AIDS* 2001; 12: 414–415.

   Assesses mortality rate in a cohort of men diagnosed with gonorrhea just before the discovery of AIDS (early 1981) through the present (end of 2000). Gay men are shown to have died at 6.5 times the rate of heterosexuals. Evidence points to AIDS as leading cause of death for gay men.

22. Potterat JJ, Brody S.   Does sex explain HIV transmission dynamics in developing countries? *Sexually Transmitted Diseases* 2001; 28: 730.

   Critiques an article that, like virtually all work coming out of Africa, fails to consider modes of HIV transmission other than sex. Maintains that until contaminated sharps are controlled for, assertions about sexual transmission's predominant role remain scientifically suspect. States that anomalies need to be properly investigated.

23. Gisselquist D, Rothenberg R, Potterat J, Drucker E.   Non-sexual transmission of HIV has been overlooked in developing countries *British Medical Journal* 2002; 324: 235.

   Challenges the assertion that heterosexual transmission of HIV has as large—and that use of unsterile medical equipment as small—a role as supposed by experts. First published outline of Gisselquist's main arguments.

24. Rothenberg R, Potterat J, Gisselquist D.   Concurrency and sexual transmission. *AIDS* 2002; 16: 678–680.

   Responds to a study in Africa that did not find the predicted association between HIV levels and sexual concurrency. We show that such an association does indeed exist, but only with classic bacterial STD. Proposes that this anomaly supports the view for HIV transmission other than sex (e.g., unsafe medical practices).

25. Gisselquist D, Potterat JJ, Epstein P, Vachon F, Minkin SF.   AIDS in Africa. *The Lancet* 2002; 360: 1422–1423.

   Critiques Lancet's 5-part series on AIDS in sub-Saharan Africa for focusing exclusively on heterosexual transmission and ignoring-dismissing parenteral exposures. Outlines, in skeletal form, evidence pointing to its probable importance and thus concludes that HIV interventions must include strongly supported "safe health care" components.

257

26. Potterat JJ, Brody S. HIV epidemicity in context of STI declines: a telling discordance. *Sexually Transmitted Infections* 2002; 78: 467.

http://sti.bmjjournals.com/cgi/reprint/78/6/467.pdf

Points out that the anomaly between the contradictory epidemic trajectories of HIV and STD in Zimbabwe during the 1990s is evidence that transmission vectors other than sex—not studied by the article's authors—should be seriously investigated as a source of HIV transmission in Africa.

27. Gisselquist D, Potterat JJ. Uncontrolled Herpes Simplex Virus-2 as a co-factor in HIV transmission. *Journal of Acquired Immune Deficiency Syndromes* 2003; 33: 119–120.

Challenges the emerging hypothesis that genital herpes is a major co-factor for the heterosexual transmission of HIV in developing countries, since studies which claim this association have not controlled for parenteral confound (i.e., patients with lesions being treated at STD clinics where contaminated medical procedures may be transmitting HIV).

28. Gisselquist D, Potterat J, Rothenberg R, Drucker E, Brody S, Brewer D, Minkin S. Examining the hypothesis that sexual transmission drives Africa's AIDS epidemic. *AIDScience* 2003; 3: 10 (10 June): http://www.aidscience.org/Articles/AIDScience032.asp

Challenges the WHO/UNAIDS response to our 4 controversial papers, which dismisses our evidence and reasserts, ex cathedra, sexual transmission as the predominant mode of HIV transmission in sub-Saharan Africa. The anomalies we detailed now require that the sexual transmission hypothesis be substantiated, not simply asserted using circumstantial, indirect, or ecologic evidence.

29. Brody S, Gisselquist D, Potterat JJ, Drucker ED. Health care transmission of HIV in South African children. *AIDScience*: 2003: 3: 14 (15 July).

http://www.aidscience.org/Articles/AIDScience035.asp

Briefly recapitulates findings of the South African national HIV serosurvey conducted in 2002.

30. Potterat JJ, Brewer DD, Rothenberg RB, Muth SQ, Brody S. HIV and hepatitis C epidemics in Africa: continuing the debate. *AIDScience* 2003; 3: 19 (16 October).

http://aidscience.org/Articles/AIDScience038.asp

Reply to article in Nature claiming that lack of parallel transmission between HIV and hepatitis-C in Africa disproves the iatrogenic hypothesis advanced by Gisselquist and colleagues. Article shows that the two viruses are not transmitted the same way: hepatitis-C is not efficiently transmitted intramuscularly, while HIV is. Also details the relative insensitivity of hepatitis-C tests (disappearance of antibody in many HIV positive patients, frequent transience of primary infection and other testing artifacts).

31. Rothenberg R, Potterat JJ, Brewer D. The case against sexual transmission of HIV. *International Journal of STD & AIDS* 2003; 14: 784–786.

Reply to a letter criticizing our view that sexual transmission is an inadequate explanation for the HIV epidemics in Africa and other poor countries. Critics are challenged to construct an epidemiologic model, using penile-vaginal transmission only, that can reproduce the epidemic curves observed in the 11 sub-Saharan countries accounting for half of HIV cases in Africa.

32. Brewer D, Rothenberg R, Potterat JJ, Gisselquist D, Brody S. HIV epidemiology in Africa: rich in conjecture, poor in data (reply to letter by Boily et al.). *International Journal of STD & AIDS* 2004; 15: 63–65.

Reply to critics of our papers, which detail the surprisingly weak empiric foundation for viewing heterosexual exposure as principal vector for Africa's HIV epidemics. Because critics' objections are speculative, we outline the required research designs for settling the controversy: in-depth contact tracing, with typing of HIV genetic sequences, and delineation of the conformation of sexual networks. (We note that in the only available study, viral profiles did not cluster in any way consistent within [or between] networks in Ugandan communities.) Data and evidence-based reasoning, not continual conjecture, are necessary to elucidate epidemic patterns.

33. Potterat JJ. Partner reduction for AIDS prevention: good luck (online letter). *British Medical Journal* 2004; 328.

http://bmj.bmjjournals.com/cgi/eletters/328/7444/891#57349

Criticizes article calling for "reduction of sexual partners" as key strategy to dampen HIV transmission in countries with generalized epidemics, because such a recommendation rests on ecologic, rather than direct, evidence of what is driving epidemics in these countries. Hard data, not insights, are needed to guide efficacious HIV prevention efforts.

34. Potterat JJ, Gisselquist D, Brody S. Still not understanding the uneven spread of HIV within Africa. *Sexually Transmitted Diseases* 2004; 31: 365.

Points out that, after 20 years of HIV epidemiology in sub-Saharan Africa, researchers have not identified even a single sexual variable that is an important personal risk for HIV acquisition and that is consistently higher in communities with higher HIV prevalence. This negative finding is important because it indicates that a substantial amount of HIV transmission is not due to sex. Also asks researchers in Tanzania to release their data on medical injections and HIV incidence.

35. Gisselquist D, Potterat JJ, Brody S. Response: Debate about iatrogenic HIV transmission should not be a pretext for inaction (Clinical Debate). *International Journal of STD & AIDS* 2004; 15: 623–625.

Response to critics who claim that we selected evidence to support the iatrogenic hypothesis (without providing any that we missed!). Among other details, we challenge the assertion that Uganda's decline in HIV incidence during the 1990s was caused by changes in sexual behaviors, for this claim does not weigh the changes in medical safety precautions implemented in the 1990s.

36. Gisselquist D, Potterat JJ. HIV transmission dynamics in Africa: still a major matter to resolve—authors' reply. *International Journal of STD & AIDS* 2004; 15: 710–711.

Reply to critics who plea for a return to the orthodox view that medical injections are not a "major" cause of HIV transmission in poor countries. We ask: how "major" does the attributable fraction have to be before implementing safe health care and warning the public?

37. Gisselquist D, Potterat JJ. Request for disclosure of available data associating HIV with medical injections (published January 5 2005).

http://uqconnect.net/signfiles/Archives/SIGN-POST00269.txt

Bluntly reiterates our multifarious (and ignored) requests for researchers in sub-Saharan Africa to fully report data associating medical injections with HIV incidence. Specifically, we request data from research teams in Mwanza, Masaka, and Rakai and we identify their funding agencies.

38. Brody S, Potterat JJ. HIV epidemiology in Africa: weak variables and tendentiousness generate wobbly conclusions. *Public Library of Science Medicine* 2005 May; 2 (5): 458–460.

http://www.plosmedicine.org/perlserv/?request=read-response&doi=10.1371/journal.pmed.0020037

Critiques use of hastily implemented, weak variables to evaluate iatrogenic HIV transmission in Africa, especially by researchers who are invested in dismissing non-sexual means of HIV transmission and who gratuitously dismiss anomalous evidence. Shows that the authors' own evidence strongly suggests non-sexual transmission, especially for their HIV positive women.

39. Potterat JJ. Estimating female-to-male infectivity of HIV-1 in Kenya: potential threats to validity. *The Journal of Infectious Diseases* 2005; 191: 2154–2155.

Criticizes a report from Kenya for failing to collect data that are sufficiently precise to validly estimate the female-to-male HIV transmission efficiency in both uncircumcised and circumcised men. Their data should have included questions about same-sex partners, anal intercourse (with men and/or women), receiving medical care for STD symptoms, and parenteral exposures.

40. Potterat JJ. Active detection of men with asymptomatic chlamydial or gonorrhoeal urethritis. *International Journal of STD & AIDS*; 2005: 16: 458.

Criticizes a CDC study for failing to frame its clinical findings in light of the epidemiologic literature. Recapitulates the empiric evidence overlooked by the authors, which demonstrates the pivotal role of asymptomatic men in the transmission of gonorrhea and chlamydia. Asymptomatic urethritis in men is common, accounts for half of all transmissions to women, and removal of infection from such unsuspecting carriers is associated with substantial (25%–33%) decreases in gonorrhea and chlamydia incidence. Silence = transmission.

41. Gisselquist D, Potterat JJ. Questioning Wawer et al.'s estimated rate of sexual HIV transmission from persons with early HIV infections. *The Journal of Infectious Diseases* 2005; 192: 1497–1499.

Critiques a report from the Rakai (Uganda) Community Trial, which claims a very high rate of seroconversion (0.0082 per sexual act) in initially HIV-negative couples. Rakai researchers failed to analyze potentially relevant evidence and failed to control for non-sexual exposures, especially the sharing of home medical injection equipment (common in Uganda). These oversights may account for the unusually high seroconversion rate noted.

42. Potterat JJ, Brewer DD, Brody S, Muth SQ. The protective effect of male circumcision as a faith lift for the troubled paradigm of HIV epidemiology in sub-Saharan Africa. *Public Library of Science Medicine* 2006; 3 (1), e64. DOI: 10.1371/journal.pmed.0030064

http://medicine.plosjournals.org/archive/1549-1676/3/1/pdf/10.1371_journal.pmed.0030064-L.pdf

Assesses the quality of the evidence from a prospective study of HIV incidence in South Africa that is being used to support the contention that circumcision has a substantial protective effect. Their study failed to control for non-sexual (e.g., puncturing) exposures and for anal (especially receptive) intercourse. It also failed to report some relevant data and analyses.

43. Potterat JJ, Brewer DD, Brody S. Miscarriage of HIV epidemiology in sub-Saharan Africa. *AIDS* 2006; 20: 955–956.

   Criticizes singular focus on sexual risk factors in sub-Saharan Africa and recommends no longer tolerating incomplete approaches (not considering exposures to sharps) in the assessment of HIV transmission in poor countries. "Unasked questions yield no answers."

44. Brewer DD, Potterat JJ, Brody S. Research design determines what can be known about modes of HIV transmission. *AIDS* 2006; 20: 1208–1209.

   Faults HIV researchers in India for allowing their preconceptions (that the observed positive association between HIV prevalence and exposures to medical injections is due to HIV patients seeking injections for their illness) to discount evidence supportive of iatrogenic transmission. Requests analogous analyses for sexual behavior correlates of HIV prevalence that they used for assessing association with medical injections. Reiterates need for better evidence (contact tracing of incident cases and sequencing of HIV DNA).

45. Brewer DD, Potterat JJ, Muth SQ, Roberts JM Jr. Rationale for using the term "prostitute" in scientific research. *Public Library of Science ONE* 2006; 1 (1): e60

   http://www.plosone.org/annotation/listThread.action?inReplyTo=info%3Adoi%2F10.1371%2Fannotation%2F13&root=info%3Adoi%2F10.1371%2Fannotation%2F13

   Responds to critic who objects to our using "prostitute" instead of "commercial sex worker"; we contend that "sex worker" is broadly encompassing and, therefore, undermines scientific precision.

46. Brewer DD, Rothenberg R, Potterat JJ, Muth SQ. Data-free modeling of HIV transmission in sub-Saharan Africa. *Sexually Transmitted Diseases* 2007; 34: 54–56.

   Criticizes mathematical modelers French and colleagues for using parameter estimates that are distantly related to empiric values; such procrustean modeling preordains a devoutly wished (yet invalid) conclusion: that heterosexual transmission, rather than iatrogenic exposures, drives Africa's epidemics.

47. Brewer DD, Potterat JJ, Muth SQ, Brody S. Converging evidence suggests nonsexual HIV transmission among adolescents in sub-Saharan Africa. *Journal of Adolescent Health* 2007; 40: 290–291.

   Challenges the conclusion of researchers in Zimbabwe who, faced with the finding that 41% of their 192 HIV-positive adolescent girls report no sexual exposure, suspect that the virgins lied about their sexual past. We propose that researchers investigate nonsexual (e.g., blood) exposures instead of simply dismissing the girls' self-reports as untrue.

48. Brody S, Brewer DD, Potterat JJ. Association of HIV infection with poor genital hygiene and medical treatment for prior serious illness suggests iatrogenic transmission. *Journal of Acquired Immune Deficiency Syndromes* 2007; 44 (3): 365–366.

   Offers an explanation for Meier et al.'s finding that good genital hygiene was associated with lower risk of HIV positivity in Kenyan men: that genital cleanliness reduces both the risk of infection and consequent risk of exposure to HIV-contaminated health care for infection.

49. Brewer DD, Potterat JJ, Brody S. Male circumcision in HIV prevention. *The Lancet* 2007; 369: 1597.

Comments on the 3 circumcision trials in Africa, cautioning against precipitous implementation of its recommendation (circumcise HIV-susceptible men) until confounding is more rigorously controlled for and until the protective effect (physiologic mechanism) is more clearly understood.

50. Brewer DD, Gisselquist D, Brody S, Potterat JJ. Investigating iatrogenic HIV transmission in Ugandan children. *Journal of Acquired Immune Deficiency Syndromes* 2007; 45: 253–254.

Questions Biraro et al.'s conclusion that >90% of children in their study acquired HIV vertically. Highlights data from their study that suggest iatrogenic rather than vertical transmission; requests additional analyses (especially from unreported study rounds); and suggests considering/assessing overlooked confounding factors.

51. Brewer DD, Potterat JJ, Roberts JM Jr., Brody S. Circumcision-related HIV risk and the unknown mechanism of effect in the male circumcision trials. *Annals of Epidemiology* 2007; 17:928–929.

Responds to critics of our paper in this journal who argue that our measurement of virginity and our small numbers have biased our results. We reply that measurement of sexual behavior is entirely irrelevant to the association we found between circumcision and HIV infection in adolescents, virgin or not—not to mention that our sample numbers were adequate for statistical assessment. We recommend that the mechanism for circumcision's protective effect be validly investigated.

52. Brewer DD, Potterat JJ, Gisselquist D, Dinsmore W, St. Lawrence J, Brody S. Valid evaluation of iatrogenic and sexual HIV transmission requires proof. *AIDS* 2007; 21: 2556–2558.

Critiques a study reporting a very strong relationship between medical injections and incident HIV in Uganda. Whereas the authors self-servingly dismiss its significance without proper empiric evidence, we present data to undermine their interpretation and request additional analyses (which they ignore by essentially reasserting their belief that their interpretation has to be right).

53. Brewer DD, Potterat JJ, Muth SQ, Gisselquist D, Brody S. Disconnects in presumed heterosexual HIV transmission in Malawi. *AIDS* 2008; 22: 1377–1379.

Suggests that both the "paradoxical distribution of HIV prevalence" in a Malawian sexual network and the lack of association between any measured sexual variable with HIV prevalence could be resolved by investigating unmeasured (especially blood) exposures.

54. Potterat JJ. Disease intervention specialists as a corps, not corpse. *Sexually Transmitted Diseases* 2008; 35: 703.

Responsibility for notifying sex partners of STD cases has traditionally rested with public health workers; it is shifting to the STD patient, who is now expected to bring Rx medication to exposed partners. Reminds STD program managers of the importance of retaining trained "shoe-leather" epidemiologists (contact tracers) for enhanced disease surveillance and control.

55. Potterat JJ, Brody S, Brewer DD, Muth SQ. Assessing anal intercourse and blood exposures as routes of HIV transmission in Mombasa, Kenya. *Sexually Transmitted Infections* 2008.

http://sti.bmj.com/cgi/es/sti.2007.028852v1

Suggests that an anomaly noted in a Kenyan HIV prevention trial could be resolved by considering non-sexual (blood) exposures to HIV, which the researchers failed to assess. Implications for prevention messages are mentioned.

56. Potterat JJ. Preventing HIV in young people in Africa: time to cut the Gordian knot? *British Medical Journal* 2008.

http://www.bmj.com/cgi/eletters/337/aug07_1/a506

Comments on editorial that expresses astonishment that an HIV intervention in South Africa moderately reduced herpes transmission, but had little impact on HIV. We suggest that, because herpes is sexually transmitted while HIV can be transmitted non-sexually, such studies should control for blood, in addition to sexual, exposures. This anomaly may then be resolved.

57. Brewer DD, Potterat JJ, Roberts JM Jr., Brody S. Unhygienic male circumcision procedures and HIV transmission. *South African Medical Journal* 2009; 99: 11–12.

Comments on a South African study that found no association between male circumcision status and HIV prevalence, while warning of the potential for HIV transmission from unhygienic circumcision procedures. We summarize evidence from one of our studies, which supports their conclusions and outline recommendations for confirmatory empiric studies.

58. Brewer DD, Potterat JJ, Muth SQ, Brody S. Raising the standard of evidence for determining modes of HIV transmission. *Public Library of Science ONE* 2009; 20 May.

http://www.plosone.org/annotation/listThread.action;jsessionid=BCC7129EF1BBEA22 E69F0567A0532857?inReplyTo=info%3Adoi%2F10.1371%2Fannotation%2F832b64de-37c2-4f15-a553 49c0731eb250&root=info%3Adoi%2F10.1371%2Fannotation%2F832b64de-37c2-4f15-a553-49c0731eb250

Compliments the authors for their strong study of HIV transmission patterns within Georgia State prisons and request additional detail, pointing out that the evidence presented suggests a much greater role in HIV transmission for tattooing than the authors conclude.

59. Brody S, Brewer DD, Potterat JJ, Muth SQ. Lack of association between heterosexual lifetime number of sexual partners and prevalent HIV infection: a crucial implication. *International Journal of STD & AIDS* 2010; 21:74–75.

Comments on McQuillan et al.'s failure to discuss the lack of association between black heterosexual men's lifetime number of sexual partners and HIV prevalence, a datum which supports the view that penile-vaginal intercourse is not a significant means of transmission.

60. Brewer D, Okinyi M, Potterat J. The facts about HIV infected Swazi children. *Times of Swaziland* 2009 (16 December): http://www.times.co.sz/index.php?news=12942

Corrects the misrepresentation of our empiric studies in sub-Saharan Africa reported by the British and Swazi press and suggests the way forward to assuring safe health care: rigorous, comprehensive, transparent, conflict-of-interest free, non-punitive investigations of blood-borne HIV infections.

61. Brewer DD, Potterat JJ, Muth SQ. Withholding access to research data. *The Lancet* 2010; 375: 1872.

Comments on Lancet editorial advocating data sharing in public health, despite probable obstacles, and points out that one of its authors is, ironically, part of a team that has denied us access to their data on several occasions.

62. Brody S, Potterat JJ. Assessing mental health and personality disorder in prostitute women. *Acta Psychiatrica Scandinavica* 2010; 122: 167.

Critiques a study of mental health in prostitute women that failed to assess personality disorders or to consider relevant published evidence, hence drawing inappropriate conclusions and recommendations.

63. Brewer DD, Potterat JJ, Gisselquist D, Collery S. Vaginal tenofovir gel trial results suggest substantial nonsexual HIV transmission. *WebmedCentral EPIDEMIOLOGY* 2010; 1: (12): WMC001292.

Comments on the CAPRISA 004 placebo-controlled trial of tenofovir vaginal gel which demonstrated a partial HIV acquisition protective effect in South African women. The data, however, strongly suggest that protection may be due to systemic absorption of tenofovir via the genital tract, which then would protect against either sexual and/or blood exposures.

64. Potterat JJ, Brewer DD. Age disparity between sex partners of MSM is only a marker of HIV risk. *Journal of Acquired Immune Deficiency Syndromes* 2011; 56 (1): e35.

Points out that the association between older age of gay men's partners and risk for HIV acquisition is less likely to be a risk factor than risk marker. The authors' assessment reflects mismeasurement of HIV exposure. Therefore, prevention messages should continue to focus on such direct risk factors as unprotected anal intercourse and sex between serodiscordant men.

65. Potterat JJ, Brewer DD, Brody S. Receptive anal intercourse as a potential risk factor for rectal cancer. *Cancer* 2011; 17 (14): 3284–3285. DOI: 10.1002/cncr.25909.

Presents evidence that the increase in rectal cancer in young (< 40 years) Americans during the last 25 years may well be due to a parallel increase in receptive anal intercourse and proposes that risk factor analyses of rectal cancer patients include assessment of anal sex practices.

66. Brewer DD, Okinyi M, Potterat JJ. Data trump speculation and distortion on routes of HIV transmission in sub-Saharan Africa. *International Journal of STD & AIDS* 2011; 22: 118–120.

Replies to two letters to the editor that criticized our study of horizontal HIV transmission in Kenyan and Swazi children. Clarifies methods and data presented in original article and, especially, presents stronger evidence than heretofore provided for how common unsafe health care is in Swaziland.

67. Gisselquist D, Hancock L, Potterat JJ, Brewer D. Grand jury report—suspect transmission of bloodborne viruses: Who can help to get an outbreak investigation underway? (Posted 20 April 2011). http://signpostonline.info/archives/477

    Appeal to invite the predominantly poor and black women attending an abortion clinic in Philadelphia to be tested for blood-borne infection. Non-sterile medical procedures in that clinic (and similar sub-standard health care settings) may help explain the high HIV infection rates in such women.

68. Brewer DD, Potterat JJ. Accumulated evidence of substantial iatrogenic HIV transmission ignored and mischaracterized. *Journal of the International AIDS Society* 2011.

    http://www.jiasociety.org/content/14/1/33/comments#531688.

    Critiques a JIAS article defending concurrency as the sexual behavior pattern most responsible for the generalized HIV epidemics in Africa. Defenders of concurrency overlook or discount plausible evidence pointing to substantial non-sexual HIV transmission in poor countries.

69. Gisselquist D, Potterat JJ, St Lawrence JS, Hogan JD, Correa M, Dinsmore W, Muth SQ. Repeating a plea for better research and evidence. *International Journal of STD & AIDS* 2011; 416–417.

    Replies to a critique of our article that misses our point—which is that the available evidence for HIV transmission in Africa is not sufficiently reliable to effectively guide prevention efforts. The need is clearly for higher quality, field-based evidence, such as the tracing of HIV infections.

70. Potterat JJ. 2010 European guideline for Chlamydia trachomatis infections: recommendation for partner notification look-back periods. *International Journal of STD & AIDS* 2011; 22: 615.

    Points out that the 2010 Chlamydia Guidelines erroneously report that empiric data are not available to recommend specific contact tracing "look back" periods, and refers readers to correct references.

71. Potterat JJ, Brewer DD, Gisselquist D, Brody S. Blood exposures ignored in racial disparities in HIV prevalence. *American Journal of Reproductive Immunology* 2011; 66: 249. DOI: 10.1111/j.1600-0897.2011.01061.x

    Comments on article calling for exploration of biological reasons for racial disparities in HIV prevalence, but which fails to consider likely confounding due to nonsexual HIV transmission.

72. Brewer DD, Potterat JJ, Brody S. Comprehensive assessment of blood and sexual exposures needed for rigorous investigation of HIV transmission. *AIDS Research and Human Retroviruses* 2012; 28: 435–436. DOI: 10.1089/AID.2011.0237

    Urges researchers in Uganda to re-interview all their patients who have phylogenetically similar viruses for both sexual and nonsexual risk factors, to determine which patients are linked by which mode of HIV transmission.

73. Potterat JJ, Brewer DD, Gisselquist D, Brody S. Sexual behavior, HIV and South African youth. *Journal of Adolescent Health* 2012; 50: 207–208.

Suggests that the substantial differences in HIV prevalence noted between South African and North American youths may be caused by differing modes of transmission and that such differences should be empirically investigated.

74. Gisselquist D, Potterat JJ, Class D, Collery S, Sonnabend J, St. Lawrence J, Correa M, Dinsmore W, Vachon F. An open letter to Michel Sibide, Executive Director of UNAIDS, Margaret Chan, Director-General of WHO, and Jim Kim, President of the World Bank. SIGNPOST 24 October 2012 (Post # 0672). http://tinyurl.com/9yw3nmr

Calls attention to international agencies of findings from recent surveys in Africa indicating HIV transmission via skin-piercing procedures in health and cosmetic care. Recommends that African public be specifically warned about often overlooked blood-borne transmission risks.

75. Potterat JJ. Are immature psychological defense mechanisms recently associated with junk food, alcohol, and television also associated with age? *Psychiatry Research* 2013; 210: 1326.

Requests that the authors of a recently published study in Psychiatry Research, who did not control for age (the possibility that with greater age comes greater maturity), newly examine their data using partial correlation analysis to assess association.

II. Letters I Authored or Co-authored
Rejected for Publication by the Editors

1. Potterat JJ. Free care for sexually transmitted diseases. *The New England Journal of Medicine* (1982).

2. Potterat JJ. AIDS, homosexual lifestyle, and premature aging of the immune system. *The New England Journal of Medicine* (1984).

3. Potterat JJ. Retroviral infection in animals: soliciting a review article for medical doctors. *The New England Journal of Medicine* (1987).

4. Potterat JJ. Laboratory assistants as unsung heroes. *Scientific American* (1988).

5. Potterat JJ. HIV patients and personal responsibility. *TIME Magazine* (1993).

6. Potterat JJ, Woodhouse DE. Risk behavior, risk group, risk space? *American Journal of Public Health* (1993).

7. Potterat JJ. Low HIV prevalence: let us praise prevention programs or network structure? *Journal of the American Medical Association* (1995).

8. Potterat JJ, Reynolds JU. Safer-sex truths. *The New York Times* (1996).

9. Potterat JJ. Safer-sex can kill you? *The New Yorker* (1999).

10. Potterat JJ. Looking for nosocomial HIV transmission. *Science* (2001).

11. Gisselquist D, Potterat J, Rothenberg R. The HIV epidemic in transition. *American Journal of Public Health* (2001).

12. Gisselquist DP, Potterat JJ. Ignoring nonsexual risks for HIV among adolescents in Zimbabwe. *AIDS* (2003).

13. Gisselquist D, Potterat JJ, Brody S, Vachon F. Le sexe ou les seringues? *Jeune Afrique* (2003).

14. Brody S, Potterat JJ. AIDS in Africa: looking ahead, and back, to the future. *Nature Medicine* (2003).

15. Gisselquist D, Potterat J, Brewer D, Brody S, Muth S, Perrin L. HIV and Hepatitis-C transmission in Africa: continuing the debate. *Nature* (2003).

16. Potterat JJ. Why Africa? *Discover* (2004).

17. Rothenberg R, Potterat JJ, Brewer D, Brody S. The need for direct evidence about HIV-1 transmission in Africa. *The Lancet* (2004).

18. Potterat JJ. HIV incidence reduction in Uganda. *Science* (2004).

19. Potterat JJ, Gisselquist D, Rothenberg RB. Controlling controlled trials of STD treatment for HIV. *Journal of the American Medical Association* (2004).

20. Gisselquist D, Rothenberg R, Potterat J. Call for broadened research into risks for HIV transmission during medical care in sub-Saharan Africa. *The Lancet* (2004).

21. Potterat JJ. Concurrent sexual partnerships have not explained Africa's high HIV prevalence. *The Lancet* (2004).

22. Brody S, Potterat JJ. Anal intercourse and bridging vectors for HIV transmission in Senegal. *AIDS* (2005)

23. Brewer DD, Potterat JJ, Brody S. Inverting the hierarchy of evidence for HIV transmission in Zimbabwe. *Science* (2006).

24. Brody S, Potterat JJ. Further ecologic evidence suggestive of health care transmission of HIV in Africa: the anomalies continue to mount. *International Journal of STD & AIDS* (2005) and *BioMed Public Health Central* (2005).

25. Potterat JJ, Brody S. Critiquing epidemiology in sub-Saharan Africa: breaking the silence. *The New England Journal of Medicine* (2005) and the *Journal of the American Medical Association* (2005).

26. Gisselquist D, Potterat JJ, Okwuosah A. Assessing information on risks for iatrogenic HIV transmission in sub-Saharan Africa: implications for safer obstetric and gynecological care. *British Journal of Obstetrics & Gynaecology* (2005).

27. Gisselquist D, Okwuosa A, Potterat J. Planning to ensure reliably sterile procedures during obstetrics and gynecological care in sub-Saharan Africa: what information is available and what is required? *Bulletin of the World Health Organization* (2005).

28. Gisselquist D, Potterat JJ. Risks of HIV transmission to and from prostitute women during health care in sub-Saharan Africa and Thailand. *Sexually Transmitted Diseases* (2005)

29. Brewer DD, Potterat JJ, Brody S. Iatrogenic transmission ignored in research on malaria-HIV link. *Science* (2006).

30. Potterat JJ. Reassessing HIV transmission? *Science* (2008).

31. Potterat JJ, Brody S. Anal intercourse in Africa. *The Lancet* (2009).

32. Potterat JJ. Fighting AIDS with circumcision. *The New York Times* (2010).

III. Published Letters to the Editor
Authored by Other Members of Our Informal Group

33. Brody S. Heterosexual transmission of HIV. *New England Journal of Medicine* 1994; 331: 1718.

34. Brody S. Incidence of HIV decreases because of nature of epidemics. *British Medical Journal* 1996; 312: 125.

35. Brody S. Risk factors for HIV-1 seroconversion may not be what they seem. *Journal of the American Medical Association* 1996; 275: 1543.

36. Brody S. Continued lack of evidence for transmission of human immunodeficiency virus through vaginal intercourse: a reply to Carey and Kalichman. *Archives of Sexual Behavior* 1996; 25: 329-337.

37. Brody S. Questioning the validity of self-reported heterosexual HIV transmission. *American Journal of Public Health* 1996; 86: 1172.

38. Brody S. Sex, lies, and genitourinary medicine: a reply to Dr. Hudson. *International Journal of STD & AIDS* 1996; 7: 305–306.

39. Brody S. Decline in HIV infections in Thailand. *New England Journal of Medicine* 1996; 335: 1998.

40. Gisselquist D. Risk factors for HIV among northern Thai women: testing hypotheses or repeating assumptions. *Journal of the Acquired Immune Deficiency Syndromes* 2001; 27: 414–415.

41. Gisselquist D. Unexplained high HIV-1 incidence in a cohort of Malawi men. *Sexually Transmitted Diseases* 2003; 30: 183–184.

42. Gisselquist D. Unanswered questions about sexual transmission of HIV in Mwanza, Tanzania. *Journal of the Acquired Immune Deficiency Syndromes* 2003; 32: 349–351.

43. Brody S. Declining HIV rates in Uganda: due to cleaner needles, not abstinence or condoms. *International Journal of STD & AIDS* 2004; 15: 440–441.

44. Gisselquist D. HIV transmission through health care in sub-Saharan Africa. *The Lancet* 2004; 364: 1665–1666.

45. Gisselquist D. New information on risks for HIV transmission in Mwanza, Tanzania. *The Journal of Infectious Diseases* 2006; 194: 536–538.

46. Deuchert E, Brody S. The evidence for health-care transmission of HIV in Africa should determine prevention priorities. *International Journal of STD & AIDS* 2007; 18: 290–291.

47. Gisselquist D. Letter to editor. *Journal of Contraception* 2008.
     Doi:10.1016/j.contraception.2008.04.123

48. Gisselquist D. Avoiding reused instruments for immunizations exposes unsolved problems. *International Journal of Occupational & Environmental Health* 2009; 107–108.

49. Brody S. The unhealthy attempts by CDC and WHO to deny the importance of HIV transmission through unsafe healthcare. *International Journal of STD & AIDS* 2009; 20: 70–72.

50. Khamassi S, Oriana'o RK, Bisika T, et al. Unsafe health care in Africa: a joint statement of the research agenda. *International Journal of STD & AIDS* 2009; 20: 879–880.

51. Gisselquist D. HIV status in serodiscordant couples. *The Lancet Infectious Diseases* 2011; 11: 658–9.

52. Gisselquist D. Use of hormonal contraceptives and risk of HIV-1 transmission. *The Lancet Infectious Diseases* 2012; 12: 510.

53. Gisselquist D. 10 years later: continuing unethical and incompetent behavior by medical professionals coincides with conflict of interest, leading to millions of unexplained HIV infections. SIGNPOST 00691 (25 March 2013).

IV. Letters Authored by Other Members of our Informal Group Rejected for Publication

54. Gisselquist D. Estimating HIV transmission rates in the United States. *Journal of the Acquired Immune Deficiency Syndromes* (2004).

55. Gisselquist D, Minkin S. An appeal for studies to fully report all data relevant to estimate proportions of HIV in African adults from sexual and non-sexual transmission. *AIDS* (2004).

56. Gisselquist D. How can we know that heterogeneous human immunodeficiency virus type 1 variants during primary infection in African women are from sexual rather than parenteral exposures? *Journal of Virology* (2004).

57. Gisselquist D. Incomplete reporting of evidence concerning HIV transmission through health care in sub-Saharan Africa. *The Lancet* (2004).

58. Gisselquist D. Risks for HIV incidence in Uganda. *The Journal of the American Medical Association* (2005).

59. Gisselquist D. Testing injection equipment in Ethiopia for presence of HIV. *AIDS* (2005).

60. Gisselquist D. Evidence of non-sexual HIV acquisition during a study of male circumcision. *PLOS Medicine* (2005).

61. Brody S. HIV incidence reduction in Uganda. *Science* (2005).

62. Brewer DD. Ongoing iatrogenic HIV transmission in African children. *Pediatric Infectious Diseases Journal* (2012).

APPENDIX THREE

INDIVIDUAL & STD/HIV PROGRAM AWARDS

National Awards:

Dr. Nathan Davis Award, 1993 (John Potterat; by the American Medical Association, for "Promoting the Art and Science of Medicine and the Betterment of the Public Health").

Special Recognition Award, 2001 (John Potterat; by the American Sexually Transmitted Diseases Association, for "numerous contributions" to the STD field).

Jack N. Spencer Award, 2002 (John Potterat; by the Centers for Disease Control, for exceptional contributions to innovative, science-based STD programs, and commitment to helping people.)

Hugo Beigel Award (John Potterat, Stephen Q. Muth & Lynanne Plummer; for best article published in *The Journal of Sex Research* in 1998.)

State Awards:

P.W. Jacoe Memorial Award, 1979 (John Potterat; by the Colorado Public Health Association, for excellence in the physical sciences.)

CHAMP (Community Health Action-Motivated Person) Award, 1987 (Mrs. Jimmie Combs, RN; by the Colorado Public Health Association, for "helpful, courteous, professional service that brings credibility and respect to public health agencies".)

Roy L. Cleere Distinguished Service Award, 1992 (John Potterat; by the Colorado Public Health Association, for outstanding contribution to public health in the State.)

Florence Nightingale Award, 1993 (Helen P. Zimmerman, RN; by the Colorado Public Health Association, for "embodying the philosophy and practice of Florence Nightingale and epitomizing the art of helping people toward their optimal health".)

Lifetime Achievement Award, Colorado Public Health Association, 1996 (Dr. John B. Muth.)

P.W. Jacoe Memorial Award, 1998 (Stephen Q. Muth; by the Colorado Public Health Association, for technical innovation in public health.)

Lillian Wald Award 1999, (Lynanne Plummer, RN; by the Colorado Public Health Association, for exemplary public health nursing leadership, initiative, and resourcefulness.)

Lifetime Achievement Award, Colorado Public Health Association, 2000 (John Potterat.)

CHAMP (Community Health Action-Motivated Person) Award, 2001 (Helen Zimmerman-Rogers; by the Colorado Public Health Association, for "helpful, courteous, professional service that brings credibility and respect to public health agencies".)

Local Awards:

Pikes Peak Advertising Federation Award (John Potterat; First Place for VD spot ads for KKFM radio, 1973.)

BOH Award, 1979 (To STD Program staff; by local Board of Health, for excellent STD control—award suggested by the Centers For Disease Control & Colorado State Health Dept.)

Pike's Peak Summit Masters Award, 1998 (John Potterat & Lynanne Plummer; for service to local gay communities.)

Leadership Award, 1999 (John Potterat; by the El Paso County Health Dept.)

Exemplary Service Award, 1999 (To the STD/HIV staff; by the El Paso County Health Dept. for overall programs excellence.)

Distinguished Alumnus Award, 2000 (John Potterat; Santa Monica High School, California; for Science.)

Award of Excellence, 2000 (Lynanne Plummer; by the Southern Colorado AIDS Project.)

Community Service Award 2000 (Helen Zimmerman-Rogers; by the El Paso County Health Dept.)

Team Efforts Hepatitis-A Award 2000 (Helen Zimmerman-Rogers; by the El Paso County Health Dept.)

Outstanding Service Award, 2002 (Lynanne Plummer; by the Southern Colorado AIDS Project.)

Special Recognition:

Eponym for concept in STD/HIV epidemiology ("Potterat structures").

APPENDIX FOUR

CONFERENCE PRESENTATIONS & ABSTRACTS
(In chronological order, presenter in bold type)

1. **Potterat JJ**. The casefinding effectiveness of a self-referral system for gonorrhea: a preliminary report. *National VD Conference*, San Diego, CA September 1977.

2. Potterat JJ, Phillips L, Rothenberg R, **Darrow WW**. Female prostitutes in Colorado Springs: a case-control pilot study. *Scientific Study of Social Problems (SSSP) Conference*, Phoenix, AZ, 26 August 1979.

3. **Potterat JJ**, Phillips L, Rothenberg RB, Darrow WW. Gonorrhea pelvic inflammatory disease: case-finding observations. *International Symposium on Pelvic Inflammatory Disease*, Atlanta, GA, April 1980.

4. Potterat JJ, **Rothenberg RB**, Woodhouse DE, Muth JB, Pratts CI. Gonorrhea as a social disease: empirical demonstration of the core group hypothesis. *5th International Society for STD Research Conference*, Seattle, WA, 3 August 1983.

5. **Rothenberg RB**, Potterat JJ. Temporal and social aspects of gonorrhea transmission: the force of infectivity. *6th International Society for STD Research Conference*, Brighton, England, August 1985.

6. **Darrow W**, Cohen J, French J, Gill P, Sikes K, Witte J, Potterat JJ, et al. Multicenter study of antibodies to HIV in American prostitutes. *III International Conference on AIDS*, Washington DC, June 1987.

7. **Darrow WW**, Bigler W, Deppe D, French J, Gill P, Potterat J, Ravenholt O, Schable C, Sikes K, Wofsy C. HIV antibody in 640 U.S. prostitutes with no evidence of intravenous (IV)-drug abuse. *IV International Conference on AIDS*, Stockholm, Sweden, June 1988.

8. **Khabbaz RF**, Darrow WW, Hartley MT, Witte J, Cohen JB, French J, Gill PS, Potterat J, et al. Seroprevalence and risk factors for HTLV-I-II infection among female prostitutes in the United States. *IV International Conference on AIDS*, Stockholm, Sweden, June 1988, Abstract # 4042.

9. **Woodhouse D**, Potterat J, Klovdahl A, Darrow W, Muth S, Muth J. Social networks in the transmission of HIV infection. *VI International Conference on AIDS*, San Francisco, CA, June 1990, Abstract S.C. 679.

10. Muth S, Klovdahl A, **Woodhouse D**, Potterat J. Protection of confidential data in HIV networks research. *VI International Conference on AIDS*, San Francisco, CA, June 1990.

11. **Darrow WW**, [Cohen JB, Wofsy C, French J, Gill P, Potterat J, Reich R, Sikes RK, Witte J] & the Collaborative Group. Reliability and validity of self-reported behaviors: implications for national and international studies. *VI International Conference on AIDS*, San Francisco, CA, June 1990.

12. **Klovdahl AS**, Potterat J, Woodhouse D, Muth J, Muth S, Darrow WW. HIV infection in an urban social network: a progress report. *XIth International Social Networks Conference*, Tampa, Florida, February 1991.

13. **Darrow W**, Boles J, Cohen JB, Elifson K, Potterat J, Schnell D, Woodhouse D. HIV seroprevalence trends in female prostitutes, United States: 1986–1990. *VII International Conference on AIDS*, Florence, Italy, June 1991.

14. **Woodhouse D**, Potterat J, Klovdahl A, Muth S, Muth J, Darrow W. HIV infection within networks of prostitute women and intravenous drug users. *VII International Conference on AIDS*, Florence, Italy, June 1991, Abstract W.C. 100.

15. **Potterat JJ**. Partner notification for HIV. *First Sino-American HIV Symposium*, People's Republic of China, Beijing, November 1991.

16. **Klovdahl AS**, Potterat JJ, Woodhouse DE, Muth JB, Muth SQ, Darrow W. Social Networks and infectious disease: the Colorado Springs study. *XIIth International Social Networks Conference*, San Diego, February 1992.

17. **Woodhouse DE**, Riffe L, Muth JB, Potterat JJ. Restriction of personal behavior: case studies on legal measures to protect the public health. *VIII International Conference on AIDS/III STD World Congress*, Amsterdam, The Netherlands, July 1992, Abstract PoD 5443.

18. **Potterat J**, Bethea P, Muth S, Woodhouse D, Muth J. A network-informed strategy for preventing HIV among street gang members. *VIII International Conference on AIDS/III STD World Congress*, Amsterdam, The Netherlands, July 1992, Abstract ThC 1516.

19. **Muth SQ**, Woodhouse DE, Potterat JJ, Muth JB, Darrow WW. HIV infection within networks of prostitute women and injecting drug users. *VIII International Conference on AIDS/III STD World Congress*, Amsterdam, The Netherlands, July 1992, Abstract ThC 1519.

20. **Potterat JJ**. 'Socio-geographic space' and focal condom use? *Behavioral Research on the Role of Condoms in Reproductive Health*. Center for Population Research, Office of AIDS Research, National Institute of Health, Bethesda, Maryland, 10–12 May 1993.

21. **Darrow W**, Potterat J, Alegría M, Rios N, Vera M, Woodhouse D. HIV prevention for streetwalkers: are condoms enough? *IX International Conference on AIDS/IV STD World Congress*, Berlin, Germany, 6/1993, Abstract WS-C08-5.

22. **Potterat JJ**. Sexually transmitted diseases in the 1990s. *Australia & New Zealand Microbiological Societies Conference*, Sydney, Australia, July 1992. And the *10th International Society for STD Research Conference*, Helsinki, Finland, August 1993.

23. **Rothenberg RB**, Woodhouse DE, Potterat JJ, Muth SQ, Darrow WW, Klovdahl AS. Social networks in disease transmission: the Colorado Springs study. *National Institute on Drug Abuse*, Rockville, Maryland, August 1993.

24. **Potterat JJ**, Muth JB. AIDS and ethical issues. *Colorado Springs Osteopathic Foundation's 5th Annual Conference on Medical Ethics*. The Broadmoor Hotel, Colorado Springs, November 1993.

25. **Rothenberg RB**, Potterat JJ, Woodhouse DE, Darrow WW, Muth SQ, Klovdahl AS. Choosing a centrality measure: epidemiologic correlates in the Colorado Springs study of social networks. *XIVth International Social Networks Conference*, New Orleans, Louisiana, February 1994.

26. **Potterat JJ**. Contact tracing: STD prevention's sleeping giant. IUVDT (International Union against Venereal Diseases and Treponematoses) World STD/AIDS Congress 1995, Singapore, March 1995.

27. **Plummer L**, Potterat JJ, Muth SQ, Muth JB, Darrow WW. Providing support and assistance for low-income or homeless women. *Behavioral Research and Evaluation Program Targeting Communities of Color Conference*, CDC, Atlanta, GA, March 1995.

28. Potterat JJ, Rothenberg RB, **Darrow WW**, Woodhouse DE, Muth SQ, Klovdahl AS. Using knowledge of social networks to prevent HIV. *Annual Meeting of the American Sociological Association* (Networks, Norms, Community, and AIDS Thematic Session), Washington DC, 20 August 1995.

29. **Rothenberg RB**, Potterat JJ, Woodhouse DE, Muth SQ, Darrow WW, Klovdahl A. Social network dynamics and HIV transmission. *National Academy of Sciences, Institute of Medicine*, Washington, DC, July 1995. And the *Annual Meeting of the American Public Health Association*, San Diego, CA, October 1995. And the *XVIth International Social Networks Conference*, Charleston, South Carolina, February 1996.

30. **Potterat JJ**, Muth SQ, Muth JB. 'Partner notification' early in the AIDS era: misconstruing contact tracers as bedroom police. *Future Directions in Partner Notification: Policy, Practice, and Research Conference*, CDC, Atlanta, GA, October 1996. And the *Tenth Annual Texas HIV/STD Conference*, Austin, Texas, July 1997.

31. Zimmerman-Rogers H, **Potterat JJ**, Muth SQ, Bonney MS, Green DL, Taylor JE, White HA. Establishing efficient interview periods for chlamydia patients. *12th International Meeting of the International Society for STD Research/ International Union against Venereal Diseases and Treponematoses*, Seville, Spain, October 1997, Abstract # 775.

32. Rothenberg RB, Malone S, **Muth SQ**, Potterat JJ. Social and geographic distance in HIV risk. *XVIIIth International Social Networks Conference*, Sitges, Spain, May, 1998. The *Infectious Diseases Society Meeting*, Boston, MA, 30 Sep–3 Oct, 2004, Abstract 834.

33. **Muth SQ**, Rothenberg R, Potterat J. Placing social networks in real geographic space: a tool for assessing HIV transmission and sample representativeness. *XVIIIth International Social Networks Conference*, Sitges, Spain, May 1998.

34. **Potterat J**, Rothenberg R, **Muth SQ**. Network structural dynamics & infectious disease propagation. *2nd European Conference on Methods and Results of Social and Behavioral Research on AIDS*, Paris, France, January 1998. And at: *International Union for the Scientific Study of Population's "Measurement of Risk and Modelling the Spread of AIDS"* seminar, Copenhagen, Denmark, June 1998.

35. **Rothenberg R**, Wasserheit JN, St Louis ME, Douglas JM and the Ad Hoc STD/HIV Transmission Group. Estimating the effect of treating sexually transmitted diseases (STDs) on HIV transmission. *12th World AIDS Conference*, Geneva, Switzerland, June 1998, Abstract 23369.

36. **Brewer DD**, Potterat JJ, Garrett SB, Muth SQ, Roberts Jr. JM, Rothenberg R. Comparison of direct estimate and partner elicitation methods for measuring number of sexual and injection partners. SSRN: http://ssrn.com/abstract=2548807. *126th Annual Meeting of the American Public Health Association*, Washington, DC, 11/1998.

37. **Brewer D**, Potterat JJ, Garrett SB, Muth SQ, Roberts JM, Kasprzyk D, Montano DE, Darrow WW. Prostitution and the sex discrepancy in reported number of sexual partners. *XIXth International Social Networks Conference*, Charleston, South Carolina, February 1999.

38. **Potterat JJ**, Woodhouse DE, Darrow WW, Muth SQ. Social networks of heterosexuals at high risk of HIV: The Colorado Springs Study. *IUSSP (International Union for the Scientific Study of Population) Conference on Partnership Networks and the Spread of HIV and other Infections*, Chiang Mai, Thailand, 7–10 February 2000.

39. **Potterat JJ** (Muth SQ, Rothenberg RB, Zimmerman-Rogers H, Green DL, Taylor JE, Bonney MS, White HA). Sexual network structure as indicator of epidemic phase. *Phase-specific Strategies for the Prevention, Control and Elimination of Sexually Transmitted Diseases*, Rome, Italy, October 3–6, 2000. Data Session III (4 Oct).

40. **Brewer DD**, Potterat JJ, Muth SQ, Malone PZ, Montoya PA, Green DA, Rogers HL, Plummer LA, Maldonado T, Hurlbutt S, Dorobiala D, Cox P. Randomized trial of supplementary interviewing techniques to enhance recall of sexual partners in contact interviews. *XXIIth Social Networks Conference*, New Orleans, February 2002. And the *National STD Conference*, San Diego CA, March 2002, Abstract # P107. And, in part, at the *15th International Society for STD Research Conference*, Ottawa, Canada, 28 July 2003, Abstract # 0340.

41. **Golden MR**, Hogben M, Handsfield HH, St Lawrence J, Potterat JJ, Holmes KK. Partner notification for HIV and STD in the United States: a survey of health departments in high morbidity areas. *2002 National STD Conference*, San Diego, CA, March 2002, Abstract LB7.

42. **Brewer DD**, Potterat JJ, Muth SQ, Malone PZ, Montoya P, Green DL, Rogers HL, Cox P. Randomized trial of supplementary interviewing techniques to enhance recall of sexual partners in partner notification contact interviews.   *XVth International STD Research Conference*, Ottawa, Canada, 28 July 2003, Abstract # 0340.

43. **Brewer DD**, Potterat JJ, Muth SQ. Interviewer effects in the elicitation of sexual and drug injection partners. SSRN Abstract 2552976. *24th International Social Networks Conference*, Portoroz, Slovenia, May 2004.

44. **Brewer DD**, Dudek JA (Potterat JJ, Muth SQ, Roberts Jr., JM, Woodhouse DE were added later). Extent and perpetrators of prostitution-related homicide. *Homicide Research Working Group Conference*, Ann Arbor, MI, June 2004.

45. **Brewer DD**, Potterat JJ, Muth SQ, Roberts JM Jr. Assessing the specific deterrent effect of arrest for patronizing a prostitute. *2004 American Society of Criminology* 19 November (56th Annual Meeting), Nashville, TN, Abstract RC 005. And the *2006 National Institute of Justice Conference*, 24 July 2006, Washington D.C.

46. **Wohlfeiler D**, Laumann E, Potterat J, Samuel M. Putting network theory into practice to reduce transmission of sexually transmitted diseases in California: successes and challenges. *XXVth International Social Networks Conference*, Redondo Beach, CA, 17–20 February, 2005.

47. Roberts Jr. JM, **Brewer DD**, Muth SQ, Potterat JJ. Prevalence of clients of prostitute women in North America. *2004 American Society of Criminology* 18 November (56th Annual Meeting), Nashville, TN, Abstract VO-029. And the *XXVth International Social Networks Conference*, Redondo Beach, CA, 17 February, 2005, Abstract Thurs D2.

48. **Brewer DD**, Muth SQ, Dudek JA, Potterat JJ, Roberts Jr. JM. Geographic profiles of violent clients of prostitute women and clients overall. SSRN: http://ssrn.com/abstract=2542635. *8th Annual Crime Mapping Research Conference*, September 7–10, 2005, Savannah, GA. And the *8th International Investigative Psychology Conference* ["Perpetrators, Profiling, Policy: Theory & Practice"], December 15–16, 2005, London, England)

49. **Gisselquist D**, Potterat JJ, Salerno L. Injured and insulted: women in Africa suffer from incomplete messages about HIV risks. *Gender, Survival and HIV/AIDS: From Evidence to Policy Conference*, Toronto, Canada, 7–9 May 2006.

50. **Potterat JJ**. Active detection of men with asymptomatic chlamydial or gonorrheal urethritis. *Workshop on the Current Chlamydia Epidemics in Western Societies*, University of Stockholm Mathematical Sociology Department, Stockholm, Sweden, 30 August 2007.

51. **Brewer DD**, Rothenberg R, Muth SQ, Roberts JM Jr, Potterat JJ. Agreement in reported sexual partnership dates and implications for measuring concurrency. *Current Chlamydia Epidemic in Western Societies Conference*, Department of Mathematical Sociology, University of Stockholm, Stockholm, Sweden, 30 August 2007. And the *XXVIIIth International Social Networks Conference*, St. Pete Beach, Florida, 22–27 January 2008.

APPENDIX FIVE

TIMELINE OF PROGRAM ACTIVITIES & FORMAL STUDIES

Reading this book, it may be easy to lose sight of the fact that so many activities of the Colorado Springs STD/HIV control programs occurred simultaneously. Lest the reader lose the forest for the trees, I trust that the following graph/timeline of activities clearly illustrates this fact.

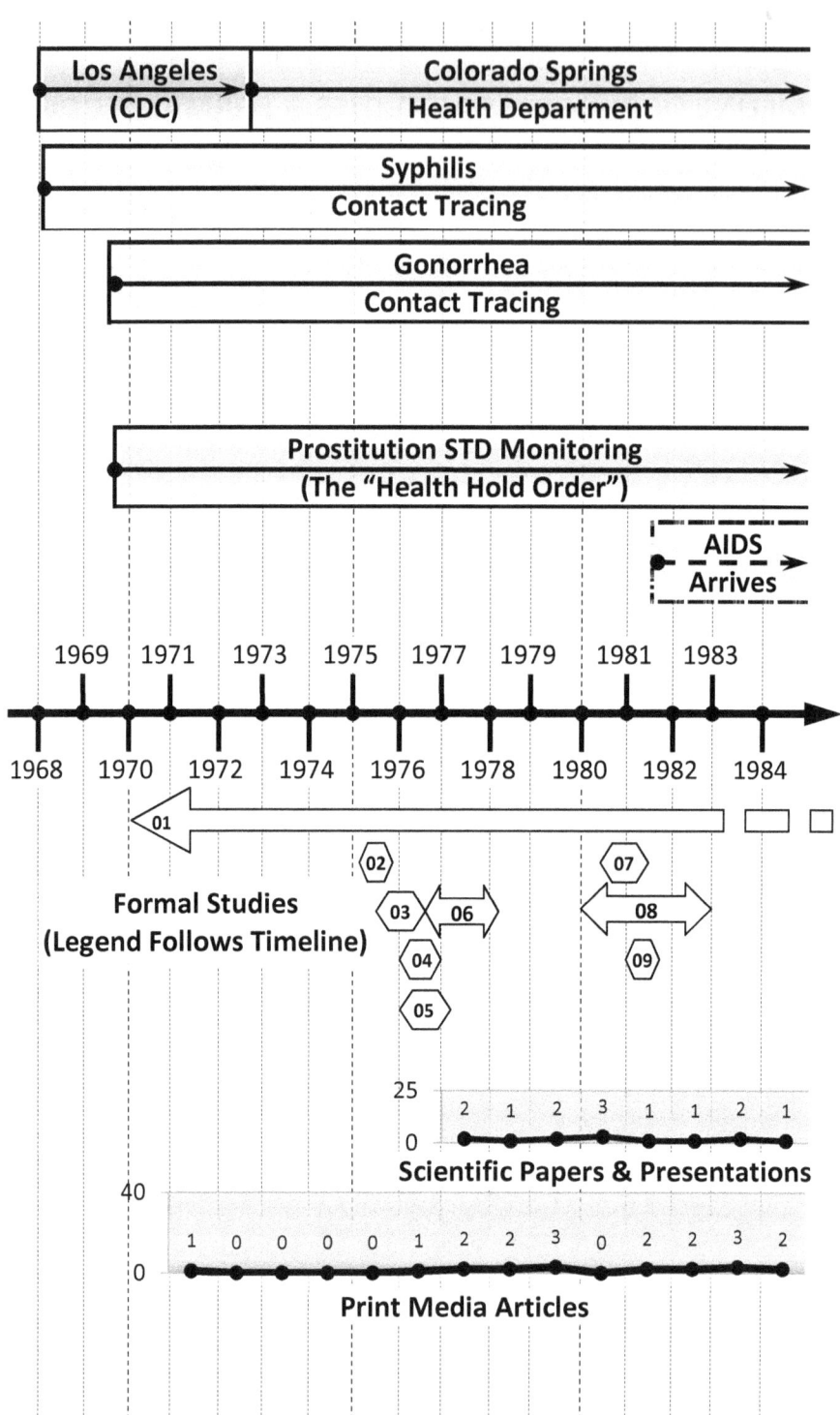

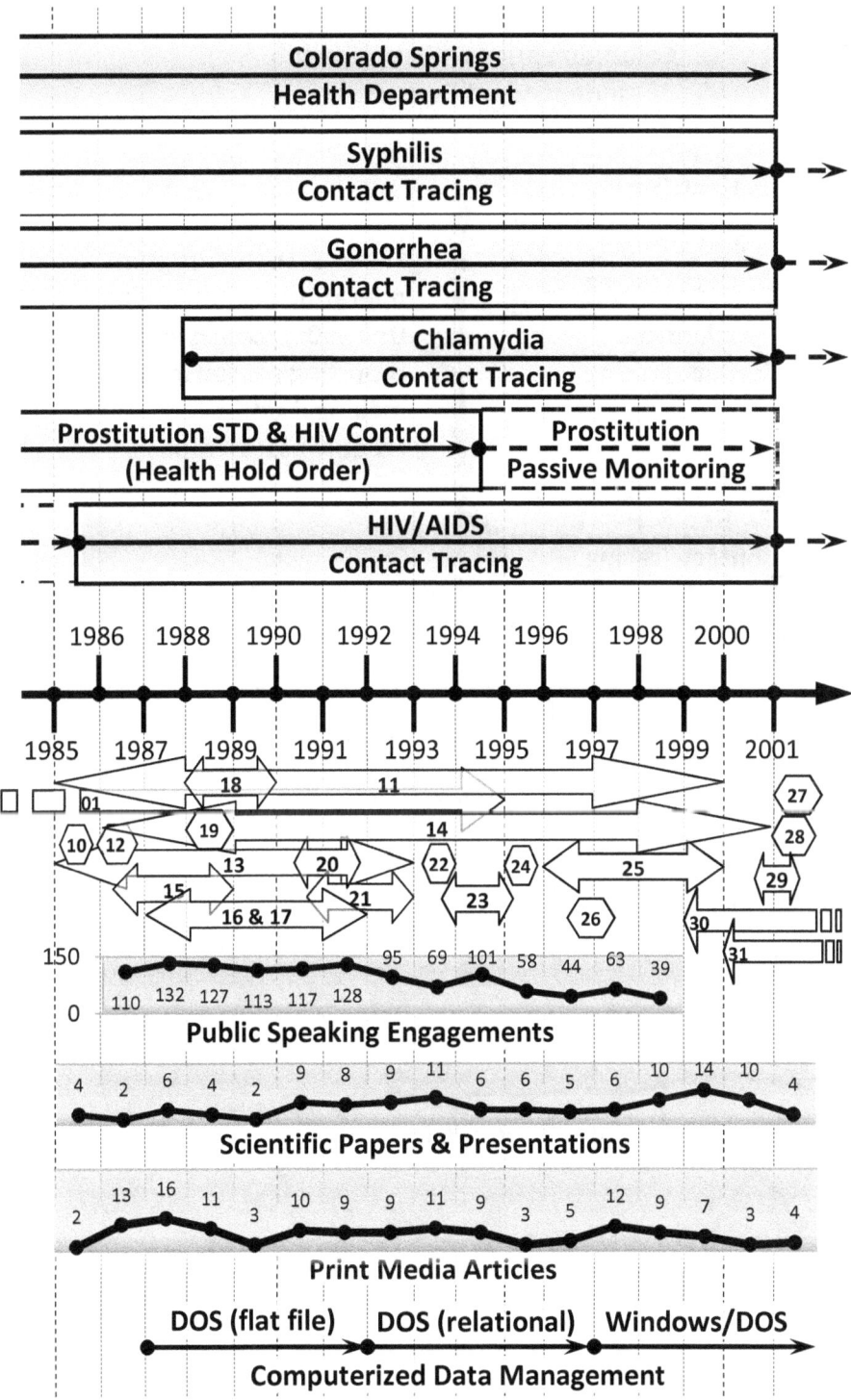

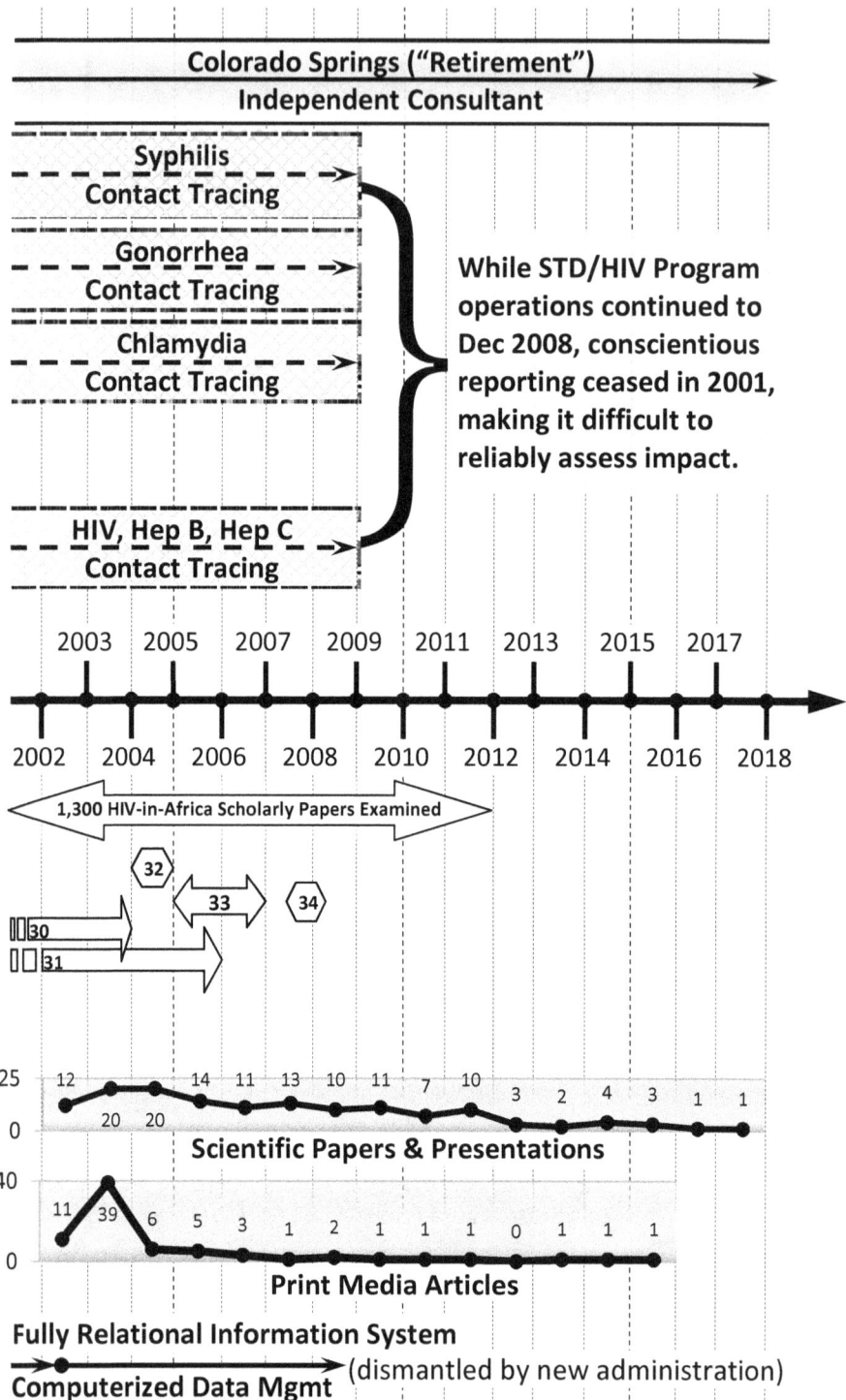

Legend for Formal Studies (1975–2008)

01	1970–1994	Impact of compulsory STD screening in prostitutes
02	Feb–Sep 1975	Evaluation of partner referral by men with gonorrhea
03	Jul 75–Aug 76	Investigation of gonorrhea in children
04	Calendar 1976	Case-control study of prostitution entry by women
05	Jan 76–Feb 77	Case-control study of prostitution impact on gonorrhea burden
06	Aug 76–Mar 78	Attributes of women associated with gonorrhea transmitters
07	Jul 80–Jun 81	Evaluation of positive case yields in women with gonorrhea
08	1980–1982	Assessing impact of saturation contact tracing on gonorrhea burden
09	Jan–Jun 1981	Identifying correlates of gonorrhea transmission
10	Jun 85	Describing sexual transmission of gonorrhea by children
11	1985–1999	Saturation HIV contact tracing and origins of local transmission
12	Nov 85–Oct 86	Improving accuracy of HIV risk factor identification in soldiers
13	1985–1992	Evidence for (lack of) HIV propagation in Colorado Springs
14	1986–2000	Applying legal measures to prevent irresponsible HIV transmission
15	May 86–1988	Assessment of blood-borne infections in local prostitutes (CDC study)
16	1987–1991	Assessing influence of network conformation on HIV transmission
17	1987–1991	Sustained street outreach for STD/HIV prevention in prostitutes
18	1988–1989	Estimating prevalence and career longevity of prostitutes in the U.S.
19	Calendar 1988	Epidemiologic differences between gonorrhea & chlamydia
20	Apr 90–Oct 91	Gang-related outbreak of penicillin-resistant gonorrhea
21	Aug 90–Dec 92	Case-control study of determinants of prostitution entry
22	May–Dec 1993	Case-control study of prostitute customers ("Johns")
23	Sep 93–Mar 95	Case-control study of rehabilitation services for prostitutes
24	Jul–Sep 1995	Assessing HIV prevalence in homeless and other marginalized persons
25	1996–1999	Chlamydia contact tracing to impact incidence & high-risk networks
26	Jul 96–Jun 97	Chlamydia contact tracing to delineate/weigh infectious periods
27	2001	Chlamydia sexual networks in Colorado Springs & Winnipeg
28	Jan 01	Estimating 20-year mortality in 1981 cohort of gay men
29	Aug 00–Jun 01	Supplementary interviewing techniques to enhance partner recall
30	1999–2003	Assessing mortality and its causes in local prostitute women
31	2000–2005	Estimating prevalence of prostitute customers ("Johns") in the U.S.
32	2004	Examination of social & geographic distances in HIV risk (1988–1992)
33	2005–2006	Assessment of deterrent effect of arrest for patronizing prostitutes
34	Aug 07–Feb 08	Study of HIV incidence correlates in Calabar (Nigeria)

REFERENCES & NOTES

PROLOGUE

1. Oldham's clever modification of the Rolling Stones's "Yesterday don't matter if it's gone..." lyric in their song, *Ruby Tuesday*. Oldham was their manager and producer (1963–1967).

CHAPTER ONE

1. Ramstedt, KM. An epidemiological approach to sexually transmitted diseases with special reference to contact tracing and screening. PhD Thesis: 1991, Department of Dermato-Venereology, University of Goteborg, Sweden.

2. Potterat JJ, Meheus A, Gallwey J. Partner notification: operational considerations. *International Journal of STD & AIDS* 1991; 2: 411–415.

3. Potterat JJ, Muth SQ, Muth JB. 'Partner notification' early in the AIDS era: misconstruing contact tracers as bedroom police, in Margolis, E (ed.): *AIDS Research/AIDS Policy: Competing Paradigms of Science and Public Policy.* Greenwich, CT, JAI Press, 1998; Vol. 6: 1–15.

4. Potterat JJ. Contact tracing's price is not its value. *Sexually Transmitted Diseases* 1997; 24: 519–521.

5. STD/HIV Control Programs, El Paso County Health Department, Colorado Springs, CO, Annual Report 1997, p. 28.

6. Potterat JJ, Muth SQ, Bethea RP. Chronicle of a gang STD outbreak foretold. *Free Inquiry in Creative Sociology* 1996; 24: 11–16.

7. Bethea RP, Muth SQ, Potterat JJ, Woodhouse DE, Muth JB, et al. Gang-related outbreak of Penicillinase-Producing *Neisseria Gonorrhoeae* and other sexually transmitted diseases—Colorado Springs, 1989–1991. *Morbidity and Mortality Weekly Report* 1993; 42 (2): 25–28.

8. Potterat JJ. 'Socio-geographic space' and sexually transmissible diseases in the 1990s. *Today's Life Science* 1992; 4 (12): 16–22, 31.

9. Potterat JJ, Spencer NE, Woodhouse DE, Muth JB. Partner notification in the control of human immunodeficiency virus infection. *American Journal of Public Health* 1989; 79: 874–876.

10. Rothenberg R, Potterat JJ. Strategies for management of sexual partners, in Holmes KK, Mardh P-A, Sparling PF, Wiesner PJ, et al. (eds.): *Sexually Transmitted Diseases.* New York, McGraw-Hill Book Co. Inc. 1984: 965–972.

11. Potterat JJ. Perspective on providing partner notification services for HIV in sub-Saharan Africa. *Journal of Retrovirology: Research and Treatment* 2014; 6: 17–21.

12. Rothenberg R, Potterat JJ. Strategies for management of sexual partners, in Holmes KK, Mardh P-A, Sparling PF, Wiesner PJ, et al. (eds.): *Sexually Transmitted Diseases* (2nd Edition). New York, McGraw-Hill Book Co. Inc. 1990: 1081–1086.

13. Rothenberg R, Potterat JJ. Partner notification for sexually transmitted diseases and HIV infection, in Holmes KK, Sparling PF, Mardh P-A, et al. (eds.): *Sexually Transmitted Diseases* (3rd Edition). New York, McGraw-Hill Book Co, Inc. 1999; 745–752.

14. Potterat JJ, Plummer L. Contact tracing in the real world: a practical partnership. *AIDS Reader* 1999; 9: 618–620.

15. Bell G, Potterat J. Partner notification for sexually transmitted infections in the modern world: a practitioner perspective on challenges and opportunities. *Sexually Transmitted Infections* 2011; 87: ii34–ii36.

16. Potterat JJ. Partner notification for HIV: running out of excuses. *Sexually Transmitted Diseases* 2003; 30: 89–90.

17. Brewer DD, Potterat JJ, Muth SQ, Malone PZ, Montoya P, Green DL, Rogers HL, Cox P. Randomized trial of supplementary interviewing techniques to enhance recall of sexual partners in partner notification contact interviews. *Sexually Transmitted Diseases* 2005; 32: 189–193.

18. Potterat JJ. Partner referral tools and techniques for the clinician diagnosing a sexually transmitted infection. *International Journal of STD & AIDS* 2007; 18: 293–296.

19. Potterat JJ. The end of laissez-faire HIV partner notification? Trust but verify. *Sexually Transmitted Diseases* 2009; 36: 463–464.

CHAPTER TWO

1. Thomas Phillip ("Tip") O'Neill was a former Speaker of the U.S. House of Representatives who said: "All politics is local", which is here paraphrased.

2. Potterat JJ, Rothenberg RB, Muth JB, Woodhouse DE, Muth SQ. Invoking, monitoring and relinquishing a public health power: the Health Hold Order. *Sexually Transmitted Diseases* 1999; 26: 345–349.

3. Henderson RH. Control of sexually transmitted disease in the United States: a Federal perspective. *British Journal of Venereal Diseases* 1977; 53: 211–215.

4. Stoffels J Jr., Wright CJ, Say BA, Carolina J, Thomas L. Pilot study: "No field follow-up", February 1973, Druid Health District, Baltimore, Maryland. Unpublished study comparing standard contact interview with self-referral for men with gonorrhea.

5. Potterat JJ, Rothenberg R. The casefinding effectiveness of a self-referral system for gonorrhea: a preliminary report. *American Journal of Public Health* 1977; 67: 174–176.

6. Yorke JA, Hethcote HW, Nold A. Dynamic and control of the transmission of gonorrhea. *Sexually Transmitted Diseases* 1978; 5: 51–56.

7. Potterat JJ, Rothenberg R, Bross DC. Gonorrhea in street prostitutes: epidemiologic and legal implications. *Sexually Transmitted Diseases* 1979; 6: 58–63.

8. Phillips L, Potterat JJ, Rothenberg RB, Pratts CI, King RD. Focused interviewing in gonorrhea control. *American Journal of Public Health* 1980; 70: 705–708.

9. Potterat JJ, Phillips L, Rothenberg RB, Darrow WW. Gonococcal pelvic inflammatory disease: case-finding observations. *American Journal of Obstetrics and Gynecology* 1980; 138: 1101–1103.

10. Potterat JJ, King RD. A new approach to gonorrhea control: the asymptomatic man and incidence reduction. *Journal of the American Medical Association* 1981; 245: 578–580.

11. STD/HIV Control Programs, El Paso County Health Department, Colorado Springs, CO, *Annual Report 1978*, p. 5. (Gonococcal PID cases declined from 130 cases at baseline in 1976, to 111 in 1977, to 85 in 1978—a 35% decrease.)

12. Wigfield AS. 27 years of uninterrupted contact tracing: the "Tyneside Scheme". *British Journal of Venereal Diseases* 1972; 48: 37–50.

13. Talbot MD, Kinghorn GR. Epidemiology and control of gonorrhea in Sheffield. *Genitourinary Medicine* 1985; 61: 230–233.

14. Washington AE, Wiesner PJ. The silent clap. *Journal of the American Medical Association* 1981; 245: 609–610.

15. Woodhouse DE, Potterat JJ, Muth JB, Pratts CI, Rothenberg R, Fogle JS. A civilian-military partnership for the reduction of gonorrhea incidence. *Public Health Reports* 1985; 100: 61–65.

16. Potterat JJ, Markewich GS, Rothenberg R. Prepubertal infections with *Neisseria gonorrhoeae:* clinical and epidemiologic significance. *Sexually Transmitted Diseases* 1978; 5: 1–3.

17. Potterat JJ, Markewich GS, King RD, Merecicky L. Child-to-child transmission of gonorrhea: report of asymptomatic genital infection in a boy. *Pediatrics* 1986; 78: 711–712.

18. Potterat JJ, Rothenberg RB, Woodhouse DE, Muth JB, Pratts CI, Fogle JS. Gonorrhea as a social disease. *Sexually Transmitted Diseases* 1985; 12: 25–32.

19. Wallace R. Traveling waves of HIV infection on a low dimensional 'socio-geographic' network. *Social Science and Medicine* 1991; 32: 847–852. (see p. 848)

20. Wallace R, Fullilove MT. AIDS deaths in the Bronx 1983–1988: spatiotemporal analysis from a sociogeographic perspective. *Environmental and Planning A* 1991; 23: 1701–1723. (See this article's Appendix)

21. Potterat JJ, Woodhouse DE, Pratts CI, Markewich GS, Fogle JS. Women contacts to men with gonorrhea: case-finding yields. *Sexually Transmitted Diseases* 1983; 10: 29–32.

22. Potterat JJ, Dukes RL, Rothenberg RB. Disease transmission by heterosexual men with gonorrhea: an empiric estimate. *Sexually Transmitted Diseases* 1987; 14: 107–110.

23. Rothenberg RB, Potterat JJ. Temporal and social aspects of gonorrhea transmission: the force of infectivity. *Sexually Transmitted Diseases* 1988; 15: 88–92.

24. Rothenberg RB, Potterat JJ. Gonorrhea surveillance: the missing links. *Sexually Transmitted Diseases* 2002; 29: 806–810.

25. Pariser H, Marino AF. Gonorrhea—frequently unrecognized reservoirs. *Southern Medical Journal* 1970; 63: 198–201.

CHAPTER THREE

1. Potterat JJ, Rothenberg RB, Woodhouse DE, Muth JB, Pratts CI, Fogle JS. Gonorrhea as a social disease. *Sexually Transmitted Diseases* 1985; 12: 25–32.

2. Centers for Disease Control: *Pneumocystis pneumonia*—Los Angeles. *Morbidity and Mortality Weekly Report* 1981; 30: 250–252.

3. Gebbie KM. The President's Commission on AIDS: What did it do? *American Journal of Public Health* 1989; 79: 868–870.

4. STD/HIV Control Programs, El Paso County Health Department, Colorado Springs, CO, *Annual Report 1985*, p. 12.

5. STD/HIV Control Programs, El Paso County Health Department, Colorado Springs, CO, *Annual Report 1999*, p. 14.

6. Redfield RR, Markham PD, Salahuddin SZ, et al.: Heterosexually acquired HTLV-III/LAV disease (AIDS-related complex and AIDS): epidemiologic evidence for female-to-male transmission. *Journal of the American Medical Association* 1985; 254: 2094–2096.

7. Potterat JJ, Phillips L, Muth JB. Lying to military physicians about risk factors for HIV infections. *Journal of the American Medical Association* 1987; 257: 1727.

8. Potterat JJ, Muth JB, Markewich GS. Serological markers as indicators of sexual orientation in AIDS-virus infected men. *Journal of the American Medical Association* 1986; 256: 712.

9. Shilts R. *And The Band Played On.* New York, St. Martin's Press (1987), p. 470.

10. Potterat JJ. The AIDS epidemic and media coverage: a critical review. *Critique: A Journal of Conspiracies* & *Metaphysics* 1987; 26: 36–38.

11. Potterat JJ. Does syphilis facilitate acquisition of HIV? *Journal of the American Medical Association* 1987; 258: 473–474.

12. Kreiss JK, Koech D, Plummer FA, et al. AIDS virus infection in Nairobi prostitutes: spread of the epidemic in East Africa. *New England Journal of Medicine* 1986; 314: 414–418.

13. Centers for Disease Control and Prevention. Racial/ethnic disparities in diagnoses of HIV/AIDS—33 states, 2001–2005. *Morbidity and Mortality Weekly Report* 2007; 56: 189–193.

14. Potterat JJ, Brewer DD, Brody S. Blind spots in the epidemiology of HIV in black Americans. *International Journal of STD* & *AIDS* 2008; 19: 1–3.

15. Peterman TA, Stoneburner RL, Allen JR, Jaffe HW, Curran JW. Risk of human immunodeficiency virus transmission from heterosexual adults with transfusion-associated infection. *Journal of the American Medical Association* 1986; 259: 55–58.

16. The CDC Collaborative Group. Antibody to Human Immunodeficiency Virus in female prostitutes. *Morbidity and Mortality Weekly Report* 1987; 36: 157–161.

17. Rosenblum L, Darrow W, Witte J, Cohen J, French J, Gill PS, Potterat J, et al. Sexual practices in the transmission of hepatitis B virus and prevalence of hepatitis Delta virus infection in female prostitutes in the United States. *Journal of the American Medical Association* 1992; 267: 2477–2481.

18. Potterat JJ. HIV infection in rural Florida women. *New England Journal of Medicine* 1993; 328: 1351–1352.

19. Potterat JJ, Brewer DD, Muth SQ, Rothenberg RB, Woodhouse DE, Muth JB, Stites HK, Brody S. Mortality in a long-term open cohort of prostitute women. *American Journal of Epidemiology* 2004; 159: 778–785.

20. Phillips L, Potterat JJ, Rothenberg RB, Pratts CI, King RD. Focused interviewing in gonorrhea control. *American Journal of Public Health* 1980; 70: 705–708.

21. Potterat JJ, Spencer NE, Woodhouse DE, Muth JB. Partner notification in the control of human immunodeficiency virus infection. *American Journal of Public Health* 1989; 79: 874–876.

22. Potterat JJ, Muth SQ, Muth JB. 'Partner notification' early in the AIDS era: misconstruing contact tracers as bedroom police, in Margolis, E (ed.): *AIDS Research/AIDS Policy: Competing Paradigms of Science and Public Policy.* Greenwich, CT, JAI Press, 1998; Vol. 6: 1–15.

23. Centers for Disease Control: Partner notification for preventing human immunodeficiency virus (HIV) infection—Colorado, Idaho, South Carolina, Virginia. *Morbidity and Mortality Weekly Report* 1988; 37: 393–396, 401–402.

24. Potterat JJ, Phillips-Plummer L, Muth SQ, Rothenberg RB, Woodhouse DE, Maldonado-Long TS, Zimmerman HP, Muth JB. Risk network structure in the early epidemic phase of HIV transmission in Colorado Springs. *Sexually Transmitted Infections* 2002; 78: Suppl 1, i159–i163.

25. Lynanne Phillips, Chris Pratts, Don Woodhouse, and I regularly visited gay bars in the Colorado Springs region as part of our "See and Be Seen" ethnographic and STD/HIV prevention approach to marginalized or hidden high-risk populations.

26. Potterat JJ. Partner notification for HIV: running out of excuses. *Sexually Transmitted Diseases* 2003; 30: 89–90.

27. Richards EP III, Rathbun KC. The role of the police power in 21st century public health. *Sexually Transmitted Diseases* 1999; 26: 350–357.

28. Rutherford GW, Woo JM. Contact tracing and the control of human immunodeficiency virus infection. *Journal of the American Medical Association* 1988; 259: 3609–3610.

29. Spencer NE, Hoffman RE, Raevsky CA, Wolf FC, Vernon TM. Partner notification for human immunodeficiency virus infection in Colorado: results across index groups and costs. *International Journal of STD & AIDS* 1993; 4: 26–32.

30. Golden MR, Hogben M, Handsfield HH, St. Lawrence J, Potterat JJ, Holmes KK. Partner notification for HIV and STD in the United States: low coverage for gonorrhea, chlamydial infection, and HIV. *Sexually Transmitted Diseases* 2003; 30: 490–496.

31. Brace NE, Zimmerman HP, Potterat JJ, Muth SQ, Muth JB, Maldonado TS, Rothenberg RB. Community-based HIV prevention in presumably underserved populations—Colorado Springs, Colorado, July–September 1995. *Morbidity and Mortality Weekly Report* 1997; 46: 152–155.

32. Woodhouse DE, Muth JB, Potterat JJ, Riffe L. Restricting personal behaviour: case studies on legal measures to prevent the spread of HIV. *International Journal of STD & AIDS* 1993; 4: 114–117.

33. Potterat JJ, Muth SQ, Stites HK. Twenty-year mortality in a 1981 cohort of homosexuals with gonorrhoea: a preliminary estimate. *International Journal of STD & AIDS* 2001; 12: 414–415.

34. Hoover DR, Munoz A, Carey V, et al. Estimating the 1979–1990 and future spread of human immunodeficiency virus type 1 in subgroups of homosexual men. *American Journal of Epidemiology* 1991; 134: 1190–1205.

35. Anonymous. Heterosexual AIDS: pessimism, pandemics and plain hard facts. *The Lancet* 1993; 341: 863–864.

36. Potterat JJ. The coming AIDS implosion. *Commentator* 1991; March/April: 19, 22.

37. STD/HIV Control Programs, El Paso County Health Department, Colorado Springs, CO, *Annual Report 1999*, pp. 11–13.

38. Potterat JJ, Woodhouse DE, Rothenberg RB, Muth SQ, Darrow WW, Muth JB, Reynolds JU. AIDS in Colorado Springs: is there an epidemic? *AIDS* 1993; 7: 1517–1521.

39. Woodhouse DE, Potterat JJ, Muth JB, Reynolds JU, Douglas J, Judson FN and the Centers for Disease Control. Street outreach for STD/HIV prevention—Colorado Springs, Colorado, 1987–1991. *Morbidity and Mortality Weekly Report* 1992; 41 (6): 94–95, 101.

40. Bethea RP, Muth SQ, Potterat JJ, Woodhouse DE, Muth JB, et al. Gang-related outbreak of Penicillinase-Producing *Neisseria Gonorrhoeae* and other sexually transmitted diseases— Colorado Springs, 1989–1991. *Morbidity and Mortality Weekly Report* 1993; 42 (2): 25–28.

41. STD/HIV Control Programs, El Paso County Health Department, Colorado Springs, CO, *Annual Report 1999*, pp. 35–36.

CHAPTER FOUR

1. Potterat JJ, Muth JB. In the shadow of AIDS: the hidden chlamydia epidemic. *The Medical Reporter* 1994; 2 (10): 8, 10–11.

2. Handsfield HH. Control of sexually transmitted chlamydial infections. *Journal of the American Medical Association* 1987; 257: 2073–2074.

3. Zimmerman HL, Potterat JJ, Dukes RL, Muth JB, Zimmerman HP, Fogle JS, Pratts CI. Epidemiologic differences between chlamydia and gonorrhea. *American Journal of Public Health* 1990; 80: 1338–1342.

4. Potterat JJ. 'Socio-geographic space' and sexually transmissible diseases in the 1990s. *Today's Life Science* 1992; 4 (12): 16–22, 31.

5. Wallace R. Traveling waves of HIV infection on a low dimensional 'socio-geographic' network. *Social Science and Medicine* 1991; 32: 847–852 (see p. 848).

6. Wallace R, Fullilove MT. AIDS deaths in the Bronx 1983–1988: spatiotemporal analysis from a sociogeographic perspective. *Environmental and Planning A* 1991; 23: 1701–1723. (see their Appendix)

7. Dylan, Bob. Title of his third studio album, released 13 January 1964 by Columbia Records.

8. Rothenberg RB, Potterat JJ, Woodhouse DE. Personal risk-taking and the spread of disease: beyond core groups. *Journal of Infectious Diseases* 1996; 174 (Supplement 2): S144–S149.

9. STD/HIV Control Programs, El Paso County Health Department, Colorado Springs, CO, *Annual Report 1982*, p. 3.

10. STD/HIV Control Programs, El Paso County Health Department, Colorado Springs, CO, *Annual Report 1992*, p. 6.

11. STD/HIV Control Programs, El Paso County Health Department, Colorado Springs, CO, *Annual Report 1999*, p. 39.

12. Potterat JJ, Zimmerman-Rogers H, Muth SQ, Rothenberg RB, Green DL, Taylor JE, Bonney MS, White HA. Chlamydial transmission: concurrency, reproduction number and the epidemic trajectory. *American Journal of Epidemiology* 1999; 150: 1331–1339.

13. Potterat JJ, Dukes RL, Rothenberg RB. Disease transmission by heterosexual men with gonorrhea: an empiric estimate. *Sexually Transmitted Diseases* 1987; 14: 107–110.

14. Zimmerman-Rogers H, Potterat JJ, Muth SQ, Bonney MS, Green DL, Taylor JE, White HA. Establishing efficient partner notification periods for patients with chlamydia. *Sexually Transmitted Diseases* 1999; 26: 49–54.

15. Starcher ET, Kramer MA, Carlota-Orduna B, Lundberg DF. Establishing efficient interview periods for gonorrhea patients. *American Journal of Public Health* 1983; 73: 1381–1384.

16. Curran JW, Schrader MV, Moyer JK, Kramer MA, Lossick JG, Brown WE. Gonorrhea in the emergency department: management, case follow-up, and contact tracing of cases in women. *American Journal of Obstetrics and Gynecology* 1980; 138: 1105–1108.

17. Phillips L, Potterat JJ, Rothenberg RB, Pratts CI, King RD. Focused interviewing in gonorrhea control. *American Journal of Public Health* 1980; 70: 705–708.

18. Potterat JJ, Phillips L, Rothenberg RB, Darrow WW. Gonococcal pelvic inflammatory disease: case-finding observations. *American Journal of Obstetrics and Gynecology* 1980; 138: 1101–1103.

19. Centers for Disease Control and Prevention. 1998 Guidelines for treatment of sexually transmitted diseases. *Morbidity and Mortality Weekly Report* 1998; 47 (RR-1).

20. Potterat JJ, King RD. A new approach to gonorrhea control: the asymptomatic man and incidence reduction. *Journal of the American Medical Association* 1981; 245: 578–580.

21. Potterat JJ. Active detection of men with asymptomatic chlamydial or gonorrhoeal urethritis. *International Journal of STD & AIDS* 2005; 16: 458.

22. Randolph AC, Washington AE. Screening for *Chlamydia trachomatis* in adolescent males: a cost-based decision analysis. *American Journal of Public Health* 1990; 80: 545–550.

23. Alexander ER. Is it cost-beneficial to screen adolescent males for chlamydia? *American Journal of Public Health* 1990; 80: 531–532.

24. Gene M, Ruusuvaara L, Mardh PH. An economic evaluation of screening for *Chlamydia trachomatis* in adolescent males. *Journal of the American Medical Association* 1993; 270: 2057–2064.

293

25. Centers for Disease Control and Prevention. Recommendations for partner services programs for HIV infection, syphilis, gonorrhea, and chlamydial infection. *Morbidity and Mortality Weekly Report* 2008; 57 (RR-9).

26. Brewer DD, Potterat JJ, Muth SQ, Malone PZ, Montoya P, Green DL, Rogers HL, Cox P. Randomized trial of supplementary interviewing techniques to enhance recall of sexual partners in partner notification contact interviews. *Sexually Transmitted Diseases* 2005; 32: 189–193.

27. Brewer DD, Garrett SB, Kulasingam S. Forgetting as a cause of incomplete reporting of sexual and drug injection partners. *Sexually Transmitted Diseases* 1999; 26: 166–176.

28. Brewer DD, Garrett SB. Evaluation of interviewing techniques to enhance recall of sexual and drug injection partners. *Sexually Transmitted Diseases* 2001: 666–667.

29. Brewer DD, Garrett SB, Rinaldi G. Free-listed items are effective cues for eliciting additional items in semantic domains. *Applied Cognitive Psychology* 2002; 16: 343–358.

30. Wasserheit JN, Aral SO. The dynamic topology of sexually transmitted disease epidemics: implications for prevention strategies. *The Journal of Infectious Diseases* 1996; 174 (Suppl. 2): S201–S213.

31. Klovdahl AS, Potterat JJ, Woodhouse DE, Muth JB, Muth SQ, Darrow W. Social networks and infectious disease: the Colorado Springs study. *Social Science and Medicine* 1994; 38: 79–88.

32. Potterat JJ, Muth SQ, Rothenberg RB, Zimmerman-Rogers H, Green DL, Taylor JE, Bonney MS, White HA. Sexual network structure as an indicator of epidemic phase. *Sexually Transmitted Infections* 2002; 78 (Suppl. 1): i152–i158.

33. Jolly AM, Muth SQ, Wylie JL, Potterat JJ. Sexual networks and sexually transmitted infections: a tale of two cities. *Journal of Urban Health* 2001; 78: 433–445.

CHAPTER FIVE

1. Potterat JJ, Rothenberg RB, Muth JB, Woodhouse DE, Muth SQ. Invoking, monitoring and relinquishing a public health power: the Health Hold Order. *Sexually Transmitted Diseases* 1999; 26: 345–349.

2. Potterat JJ, Rothenberg R, Bross DC. Gonorrhea in street prostitutes: epidemiologic and legal implications. *Sexually Transmitted Diseases* 1979; 6: 58–63.

3. Woodhouse DE, Potterat JJ, Muth JB, Reynolds JU, Douglas J, Judson FN and the Centers for Disease Control. Street outreach for STD/HIV prevention—Colorado Springs, Colorado, 1987–1991. *Morbidity and Mortality Weekly Report* 1992; 41 (6): 94–95, 101.

4. STD/HIV Control Programs, El Paso County Health Department, Colorado Springs, CO, *Annual Report 1999*, pp. 34–35.

5. Potterat JJ, Brewer DD, Muth SQ, Rothenberg RB, Woodhouse DE, Muth JB, Stites HK, Brody S. Mortality in a long-term open cohort of prostitute women. *American Journal of Epidemiology* 2004; 159: 778–785.

6. Phillips L, Potterat JJ, Rothenberg RB, Pratts CI, King RD. Focused interviewing in gonorrhea control. *American Journal of Public Health* 1980; 70: 705–708.

7. Potterat JJ, Phillips L, Rothenberg RB, Darrow WW. Gonococcal pelvic inflammatory disease: case-finding observations. *American Journal of Obstetrics and Gynecology* 1980; 138: 1101–1103.

8. Potterat JJ, Phillips L, Rothenberg RB, Darrow WW. On becoming a prostitute: an exploratory case-comparison study. *Journal of Sex Research* 1985; 21: 329–335.

9. Potterat JJ, Rothenberg RB, Muth SQ, Darrow WW, Phillips-Plummer L. Pathways to prostitution: the chronology of sexual and drug abuse milestones. *Journal of Sex Research* 1998; 35: 333–340.

10. Gray D. Turning out: a study of teenage prostitution. *Urban Life and Culture* 1973; 1: 401–425.

11. Polonsky MJ. The not-so-happy hooker: a psychological comparison between professional prostitutes and other women. *Unpublished doctoral dissertation* (1974), University of Tennessee, Knoxville.

12. Exner JE Jr., Wylie J, Leura A, Parrill T. Some psychological characteristics of prostitutes. *Journal of Personality Assessment* 1977; 41: 474–485.

13. The CDC Collaborative Group. Antibody to Human Immunodeficiency Virus in female prostitutes. *Morbidity and Mortality Weekly Report* 1987; 36 (11): 157–161.

14. Khabbaz RF, Darrow WW, Hartley MT, Witte J, Cohen JB, French J, Gill PS, Potterat J, et al. Seroprevalence and risk factors for HTLV-I/II infection among female prostitutes in the United States. *Journal of the American Medical Association* 1990; 263: 60–64.

15. Rosenblum L, Darrow W, Witte J, Cohen J, French J, Gill PS, Potterat J, et al. Sexual practices in the transmission of hepatitis B virus and prevalence of hepatitis Delta virus infection in female prostitutes in the United States. *Journal of the American Medical Association* 1992; 267: 2477–2481.

16. Darrow WW, and the Centers for Disease Control Collaborative Group for the Study of HIV-1 in Selected Women. Prostitution, intravenous drug use and HIV-1 in the United States, in Plant MA (ed.): *AIDS, Drugs, and Prostitution*. London, Routledge 1990: 18–40.

17. Goldstein PJ. Prostitution and Drugs. Lexington, MA: Lexington Books (1979).

18. James J. Ethnography and social problems. In: Weppner RS (ed.): *Street Ethnography: Selected Studies of Crime and Drug use in Natural Settings*; vol. 1: 179–200. Beverly Hills, CA: Sage Publications, 1977.

19. Silbert MH, Pines AM, Lynch T. Substance abuse and prostitution. *Journal of Psychoactive Drugs* 1982; 14:193–197.

20. De Schampheleire D. MMPI characteristics of professional prostitutes: A cross-cultural replication. *Journal of Personality Assessment* 1990; 54: 343–350.

21. Simon PM, Morse EV, Osovsky HJ, Balson PM, Gaumer HR. Psychological characteristics of a sample of male prostitutes. *Archives of Sexual Behavior* 1992; 21: 33–44.

22. Brody S, Potterat JJ, Muth SQ, Woodhouse DE. Psychiatric and characterological factors relevant to excess mortality in a long-term cohort of prostitute women. *Journal of Sex & Marital Therapy* 2005; 31: 97–112.

23. Plummer L, Potterat JJ, Muth SQ, Muth JB, Darrow WW. Providing support and assistance for low-income or homeless women. *Journal of the American Medical Association* 1996; 276: 1874–1875.

24. Turner CF, Miller HG, Moses LE (eds.). *AIDS: Sexual Behavior and Intravenous Drug Use.* National Academy Press 1989. Washington DC.

25. Potterat JJ, Woodhouse DE, Muth JB, Muth SQ. Estimating the prevalence and career longevity of prostitute women. *Journal of Sex Research* 1990; 27: 233–243.

26. Potterat JJ, Dukes RL, Rothenberg RB. Disease transmission by heterosexual men with gonorrhea: an empiric estimate. *Sexually Transmitted Diseases* 1987; 14: 107–110.

27. Sudman S, Sirken MG, Cowan CD. Sampling rare and elusive populations. *Science* 1988; 240: 994–995.

28. Michael RT, Laumann EO, Gagnon JH, Smith TW. Numbers of sex partners and potential risk of sexual exposure to Human Immunodeficiency Virus. *Morbidity and Mortality Weekly Report* 1988; 37: 565–568.

29. Ward H, Day S, Weber J. Risky business: health and safety in the sex industry over a 9-year period. *Sexually Transmitted Infections* 1999; 75: 340–343.

30. Brewer D, Potterat JJ, Garrett SB, Muth SQ, Roberts JM, Kasprzyk D, Montano DE, Darrow WW. Prostitution and the sex discrepancy in reported number of sexual partners. *Proceedings of the National Academy of Sciences* 2000; 97: 12385–12388.

31. Brewer DD, Potterat JJ, Muth SQ, Roberts JM Jr. Rationale for using the term "prostitute" in scientific research. *Public Library of Science ONE* 2006; 1 (1): e60. http://www.plosone.org/annotation/listThread.action?root=1573

32. Brewer DD, Roberts JM Jr., Muth SQ, Potterat JJ. Prevalence of male clients of street prostitute women in the United States. *Human Organization* 2008; 67 (3): 346–356.

33. Brewer DD, Muth SQ, Potterat JJ. Demographic, biometric, and geographic comparison of clients of prostitutes and men in the US general population. *Electronic Journal of Human Sexuality* 2008; Vol. 11. http://www.ejhs.org/volume11/brewer.htm

34. Brewer DD, Dudek JA, Potterat JJ, Muth SQ, Roberts JM Jr., Woodhouse DE. Extent, trends, and perpetrators of prostitution-related homicide in the United States. *The Journal of Forensic Sciences* 2006; 51 (5): 1101–1108.

35. Brewer DD, Potterat JJ, Muth SQ, Roberts JM Jr. A large specific deterrent effect of arrest for patronizing a prostitute. *Public Library of Science ONE* 2006; 1 (1): e60. http://journals.plos.org/plosone/article?id=10.1371/journal.pone.0000060

CHAPTER SIX

1. Klovdahl AS. Social networks and the spread of infectious diseases: the AIDS example. *Social Science and Medicine* 1985; 21: 1203–1216.

2. Centers for Disease Control. A cluster of Kaposi's sarcoma and *Pneumocystis carinii* pneumonia among homosexual male residents of Los Angeles and Orange counties. *Morbidity and Mortality Weekly Report* 1982; 31: 305–307.

3. Auerbach DM, Darrow WW, Jaffe HW, Curran JW. Cluster of cases of the acquired immune deficiency syndrome: patients linked by sexual contact. *American Journal of Medicine* 1984; 76: 487–492. [Further detail is available in: Darrow WW. AIDS: Socioepidemiologic responses to an epidemic. In Ulack R, Skinner WF (eds.) *AIDS and the Social Sciences: Common Threads.* University of Kentucky Press 1991.]

4. Freeman LC. The Development of Social Network Analysis: A study in the Sociology of Science. BookSurge LLC, North Charleston, South Carolina 2004.

5. Potterat JJ. The AIDS epidemic and media coverage: a critical review. *Critique: A Journal of Conspiracies & Metaphysics* 1987; 26: 36–38.

6. Moreno JL. *Who Shall Survive?* Washington D.C.: Nervous and Mental Disease Publishing Company, 1934.

7. Wasserman S, Faust K. *Social Network Analysis: Methods and Applications.* Cambridge University Press 1994.

8. Klovdahl AS, Potterat J, Woodhouse D, Muth J, Muth S, Darrow WW. HIV infection in an urban social network: a progress report. *Bulletin de Méthodologie Sociologique* 1992; 36: 24–33.

9. Potterat JJ, Woodhouse DE, Muth SQ, Rothenberg RB, Darrow WW, Klovdahl AS, Muth JB. Network dynamism: history and lessons of the Colorado Springs study, in Morris M (ed.). *Network Epidemiology: A Handbook for Survey Design and Data Collection.* Oxford University Press Inc., New York 2004: 87–114. http://www.oup.co.uk/isbn/0-19-926901-7

10. Woodhouse DE, Potterat JJ, Rothenberg RB, Darrow WW, Klovdahl AS, Muth SQ. Ethical and legal issues in social networks research: the real and the ideal, in Needle RH, Genser SG, Trotter II RT (eds.): *Social Networks, Drug Abuse and HIV Transmission.* National Institute of Drug Abuse Monograph No. 151 (NIH Publication No. 95-3889); 1995: 131–143.

11. Rothenberg RB, Woodhouse DE, Potterat JJ, Muth SQ, Darrow WW, Klovdahl AS. Social networks in disease transmission: the Colorado Springs study, in Needle RH, Genser SG, Trotter II RT, (eds.): *Social Networks, Drug Abuse and HIV Transmission.* National Institute of Drug Abuse Research Monograph No. 151 (NIH Publication No. 95-3889); 1995: 3–19.

12. The 14 people who contributed to the behavioral questionnaire's contents (in alphabetical order): Sabine Bartholomeyczik, Jackie Boles, Judith Cohen, Bill Darrow, Kirk Elifson, John Gagnon, Rima Khabbaz, Alden Klovdahl, Stephen Muth, Lynanne Plummer, John Potterat, Claire Sterk, Donald Woodhouse, and Constance Wofsy. And the five Project 90 interviewers were: Lynanne Plummer, John Potterat, Donald Woodhouse, Helen L. Zimmerman-Rogers, and Helen P. Zimmerman.

13. Klovdahl AS, Potterat JJ, Woodhouse DE, Muth JB, Muth SQ, Darrow W. Social networks and infectious disease: the Colorado Springs study. *Social Science and Medicine* 1994; 38: 79–88.

14. Darrow WW, Potterat JJ, Rothenberg RB, Woodhouse DE, Muth SQ, Klovdahl AS. Using knowledge of social networks to prevent human immunodeficiency virus infections: the Colorado Springs study. *Sociological Focus* 1999; 32: 143–158.

15. Potterat JJ, Rothenberg RB, Muth SQ. Network structural dynamics and infectious disease propagation. *International Journal of STD & AIDS* 1999; 10: 182–185.

16. See: http://en.wikipedia.org/wiki/Dynaflo (for origin of this word).

17. Rothenberg RB, Potterat JJ, Woodhouse DE. Personal risk-taking and the spread of disease: beyond core groups. *Journal of Infectious Diseases* 1996; 174 (Suppl. 2): S144–S149.

18. Rothenberg RB, Sterk C, Long D, Patch A, Potterat JJ, Muth SQ. The Atlanta urban networks study: a blueprint for endemic transmission. *AIDS* 2000; 14: 2191–2200.

19. Rothenberg RB, Potterat JJ, Woodhouse DE, Muth SQ, Darrow WW, Klovdahl A. Social network dynamics and HIV transmission. *AIDS* 1998; 12: 1529–1536.

20. Rothenberg RB, Potterat JJ, Woodhouse DE, Darrow WW, Muth SQ, Klovdahl AS. Choosing a centrality measure: epidemiologic correlates in the Colorado Springs study of social networks. *Social Networks* 1995; 17: 273–297.

21. Rothenberg RB. The geography of gonorrhea: empirical demonstration of core group transmission. *American Journal of Epidemiology* 1983; 117: 688–694.

22. Potterat JJ, Rothenberg RB, Woodhouse DE, Muth JB, Pratts CI, Fogle JS. Gonorrhea as a social disease. *Sexually Transmitted Diseases* 1985; 12: 25–32.

23. Rothenberg RB, Muth SQ, Malone SL, Potterat JJ, Woodhouse DE. Social and geographic distance in HIV risk. *Sexually Transmitted Diseases* 2005; 32: 506–512.

24. Zenilman JM, Ellish N, Friesia A, et al. The geography of sexual partnerships in Baltimore: applications of core theory dynamics using a geographic information system. *Sexually Transmitted Diseases* 1999; 26: 75–81.

25. Tobler WR. A computer movie stimulating urban growth in the Detroit region. *Economic Geography* 1970; 46: 234–240.

26. Muth SQ, Potterat JJ, Rothenberg RB. Birds of a feather: using a rotational box plot to assess ascertainment bias. *International Journal of Epidemiology* 2000; 29: 899–904.

27. Rothenberg R, Sterk C, Toomey KE, Potterat JJ, Johnson D, Schrader M, Hatch S. Using social network and ethnographic tools to evaluate syphilis transmission. *Sexually Transmitted Diseases* 1998; 25: 154–160.

28. Morris M, Kretzschmar M. Concurrent partnerships and transmission dynamics in networks. *Social Networks* 1995; 17: 299–318.

29. Personal communication with Dr. Alden Klovdahl on 24 November 2014.

30. Foster KC, Muth SQ, Potterat JJ, Rothenberg RB. A faster Katz status score algorithm. *Computational & Mathematical Organization Theory* 2001; 7: 275–285.

31. See Appendix One

32. Potterat JJ, Muth SQ, Bethea RP. Chronicle of a gang STD outbreak foretold. *Free Inquiry in Creative Sociology* 1996; 24: 11–16.

33. Potterat JJ, Phillips-Plummer L, Muth SQ, Rothenberg RB, Woodhouse DE, Maldonado-Long TS, Zimmerman HP, Muth JB. Risk network structure in the early epidemic phase of HIV transmission in Colorado Springs. *Sexually Transmitted Infections* 2002; 78 (Suppl. 1): i159–i163.

34. Potterat JJ, Muth SQ, Rothenberg RB, Zimmerman-Rogers H, Green DL, Taylor JE, Bonney MS, White HA. Sexual network structure as an indicator of epidemic phase. *Sexually Transmitted Infections* 2002; 78 (Suppl. 1): i152–i158.

35. Woodhouse DE, Rothenberg RB, Potterat JJ, Darrow WW, Muth SQ, Klovdahl AS, Zimmerman HP, Rogers HL, Maldonado TS, Muth JB, Reynolds JU. Mapping a social network of heterosexuals at high risk of HIV infection. *AIDS* 1994; 8: 1331–1336.

36. Jolly AM, Muth SQ, Wylie JL, Potterat JJ. Sexual networks and sexually transmitted infections: a tale of two cities. *Journal of Urban Health* 2001; 78: 433–445.

37. Chow M, Thompson SK. Estimation with link-tracing sampling designs: a Bayesian approach. *Survey Methodology* 2003; 29: 197–205.

38. Thompson SK. Targeted random walk designs. *Survey Methodology* 2006; 32: 11–24.

39. Thompson SK. Adaptive web sampling. *Biometrics* 2006; 62: 1224–1234.

40. Goel S, Salganik MJ. Assessing respondent-driven sampling. *Proceedings of the National Academy of Sciences* 2010; 107 (15): 6743–6747.

41. Felix-Medina MH, Monjardin PE. Combining link-tracing sampling and cluster sampling to estimate totals and means of hidden human populations. *Journal of Official Statistics* 2010; 26 (4): 603–631.

42. St. Clair K, O'Connell D. A Bayesian model for estimating population means using link-tracing sampling design. *Biometrics* 2011. DOI: 10.1111/j.1541-0420.2011.01631.x

43. Moody J, Adams J, Muth S, Morris M. Quantifying the benefits of link-tracing designs for partnership network studies. *Field Methods* 2012; 24: 175–193.

44. Moody J, Adams J. "To tell the truth": measuring concordance in multiply reported network data. *Social Networks* 2007; 29: 44–58.

45. Roberts JM, Brewer DD. Measures and tests of heaping in discrete quantitative distributions. *Journal of Applied Statistics* 2001; 28: 887–896.

46. Szendroi B, Csanyi G. Polynomial epidemics and clustering in contact networks. *Proceedings of the Royal Society London B Biol Sci* 2004; 271 (Suppl. 5): S364–S366.

47. Newman MEJ. A measure of betweenness centrality based on random walks. 1 Sept 2003. *ArXiv: cond-mat/0309045v1*

48. Adams J, Moody J, Morris M. Sex, drugs and race: how behaviors differentially contribute to STI-risk network structure. *American Journal of Public Health* 2013; 103: 322–329.

49. Lind PG, Gonzalez MC, Hermann HJ. Cycles and clustering in bipartite networks. *Physical Review E* 2005. DOI: 10.1103/PhysRevE.72056127.

50. Gonzalez MC, Lindt PG, Hermann HJ. Model of mobile agents for sexual interactions networks. *The European Physical Journal B* 2006; 49: 371–376.

51. Butts CT. Revisiting the foundations of network analysis. *Science* 2009; 325: 414–416.

52. Goodreau S. Assessing the effects of human mixing patterns on Human Immunodeficiency Virus-I interhost phylogenetics through social network simulation. *Genetics* 2006; 172: 2033–2045.

53. Rothenberg R, Muth SQ. Large-network concepts and small-network characteristics: fixed and variable factors. *Sexually Transmitted Diseases* 2007; 34: 604–612.

CHAPTER SEVEN

1. Potterat JJ, Muth JB, Markewich GS. Serological markers as indicators of sexual orientation in AIDS-virus infected men. *Journal of the American Medical Association* 1986; 256: 712.

2. Potterat JJ, Phillips L, Muth JB. Lying to military physicians about risk factors for HIV infections. *Journal of the American Medical Association* 1987; 257: 1727.

3. Potterat JJ. Does syphilis facilitate acquisition of HIV? *Journal of the American Medical Association* 1987; 258: 473–474.

4. Potterat JJ. HIV infection in rural Florida women. *New England Journal of Medicine* 1993; 328: 1351–1352.

5. Potterat JJ, Woodhouse DE, Rothenberg RB, Muth SQ, Darrow WW, Muth JB, Reynolds JU. AIDS in Colorado Springs: is there an epidemic? *AIDS* 1993; 7: 1517–1521.

6. Brody S, Potterat JJ. Re: "Is there really a heterosexual AIDS epidemic in the United States? Findings from a multisite validation study: 1992–1995". *American Journal of Epidemiology* 1999; 150: 429–430.

7. Potterat JJ. The AIDS epidemic and media coverage: a critical review. *Critique: A Journal of Conspiracies & Metaphysics* 1987; 26: 36–38.

8. Gisselquist DP. Estimating HIV-1 transmission efficiency through unsafe medical injections. *International Journal of STD & AIDS* 2002; 13: 152–159.

9. Potterat JJ, Brody S. Does sex explain HIV transmission dynamics in developing countries? *Sexually Transmitted Diseases* 2001; 28: 730.

10. Gisselquist D, Rothenberg R, Potterat J, Drucker E. Non-sexual transmission of HIV has been overlooked in developing countries. *British Medical Journal* 2002; 324: 235.

11. Rothenberg R, Potterat J, Gisselquist D. Concurrency and sexual transmission. *AIDS* 2002; 16: 678–680.

12. Gisselquist D, Potterat JJ, Epstein P, Vachon F, Minkin SF. AIDS in Africa. *The Lancet* 2002; 360: 1422–1423.

13. Potterat JJ, Brody S. HIV epidemicity in context of STI declines: a telling discordance. *Sexually Transmitted Infections* 2002; 78: 467.

14. Gisselquist D, Rothenberg R, Potterat J, Drucker E. HIV infections in Sub-Saharan Africa not explained by sexual or vertical transmission. *International Journal of STD & AIDS* 2002; 13: 657–666.

15. Russell S. New AIDS suspect/Researchers say reuse of needles as much to blame as sex behavior. *The San Francisco Chronicle*, 1 December 2002.

16. This initial group includes Stuart Brody, Devon Brewer, Ernest Drucker, Paul Epstein, David Gisselquist, Steven Minkin, John Potterat, Richard Rothenberg, and Francois Vachon. Others who were involved a bit later include Eric Friedman, Yvan Hutin, Savanna Reid, Lillian Salerno and last, but never least (au contraire!), Garance "Nance" Upham.

17. In alphabetical order: Brewer DD, Brody S, Drucker E, Gisselquist D, Minkin SF, Potterat JJ, Rothenberg RB, Vachon F. Mounting anomalies in the epidemiology of AIDS in Africa: cry the beloved paradigm. *International Journal of STD & AIDS* 2003; 14: 144–147.

18. Gisselquist D, Potterat J, Brody S, Vachon F. Let it be sexual: how health care transmission of AIDS in Africa was ignored. *International Journal of STD & AIDS* 2003; 14: 148–161.

19. Gisselquist D, Potterat JJ. Heterosexual transmission of HIV in Africa: an empiric estimate. *International Journal of STD & AIDS* 2003; 14: 162–173.

20. Gisselquist D, Potterat J. Confound it: latent lessons from the Mwanza trial of STD treatment to reduce HIV transmission. *International Journal of STD & AIDS* 2003; 14: 179–184.

21. Epprecht M. Heterosexual Africa: The History of an Idea from the Age of Exploration to the Age of AIDS. Ohio/Scoville: Ohio University/University KwaZulu-Natal, 2008.

22. Buve A, Carael M, Hayes RJ, et al. The multicenter study on factors determining the differential spread of HIV in four African cities: summary and conclusions. *AIDS* 2001; 15 (Suppl. 4): S127–S131.

23. Van de Perre P, Carael M, Naramba D, et al. Risk factors for HIV seropositivity in selected urban-based Rwandese adults. *AIDS* 1987; 1: 207–211.

24. Schmid G. "Meeting Agenda Change" emails of 28 February, 2 March, & 4 March 2003.

25. Hoelsscher M, Riedner G, Hemed Y, Wagner HU, Korte R, von Sonnenburg F. Estimating the number of HIV transmissions through reused syringes and needles in the Mbeya Region, Tanzania. *AIDS* 1994; 8: 1609–1615.

26. Schmid G, Buve A, Mugyeni P, et al. Transmission of HIV-1 infection in sub-Saharan Africa and effect of elimination of unsafe injections. *The Lancet* 2004; 363: 482–488.

27. Vos J, Gumodoka B, van Asten HA, Berege ZA, Dolmans WM, Borgdorff MW. Improved injection practices after the introduction of treatment and sterility guidelines in Tanzania. *Tropical Medicine & International Health* 1998; 3; 291–296.

28. Copies of these documents are available from John Potterat: jjpotterat@earthlink.net.

29. Whitworth JA, Biraro S, Shafer LA, Morison LA, Quigley M, White RG, et al. HIV incidence and recent injections among adults in rural southwestern Uganda. *AIDS* 2007; 21: 1056–1058.

30. Seguy N. Literature review of epidemiological studies estimating the risk of HIV infection associated with health care injections. 5 September 2002 (Unpublished CDC manuscript). Reported in Randerson J. WHO accused of huge HIV blunder. *New Scientist* 2003; 180 (2424): 8–9. This draft is available from david.gisselquist@yahoo.com or jjpotterat@earthlink.net.

31. Ecologic evidence is the most distant from actual transmission events and hence makes it difficult to confidently determine cause and effect. For example, concluding that the cause of HIV epidemics in Africa must be sexual transmission because cases are evenly distributed between men and women, and because the cases' age distributions are highest in the sexually active years, is an ecologic inference. Such a conclusion is not based on the stronger evidence derived from linking cases via, for example, contact tracing.

32. Viswanathan M, Lux L, Kirmeyer S, et al. Examination of Health Care Transmission of HIV/AIDS in Sub-Saharan Africa and the Caribbean Region: A Literature Review, Expert Panel, and Report. RTI Project Number: 08490.005 (Final Report: 2 January 2004).

33. Potterat John J. The enigma of HIV propagation in Africa: mainstream thought has narrowly focused on "heterosexual sex". *Social Science Research Network* 2310200 (14 August 2013). Available at SSRN: http://ssrn.com/abstract=2310200

34. Kalichman SC. *Denying AIDS: Conspiracy Theories, Pseudoscience and Human Tragedy.* Berlin: Springer Science + Business Media LLC, 2009.

35. Potterat JJ. AIDS denialism is not the same as AIDS dissent. *International Journal of STD & AIDS* 2009; 20: 515–516.

36. Safe Injection Global Network. *SIGNPOST.* Call for Articles. Post # 00123, 26 June 2002.

37. Shisana O, Simbayi L, Bezuidenhout F, et al. Nelson Mandela/HSCR study of HIV/AIDS: South African national HIV prevalence, behavioural risks and mass media: household survey 2002. *Capetown, Human Sciences Research Council* 2002.

38. Brody S, Gisselquist D, Potterat JJ, Drucker E. Evidence for iatrogenic HIV transmission in children in South Africa. *British Journal of Obstetrics & Gynaecology* 2003; 110: 450–452.

39. Gisselquist D, Potterat JJ, Brody S. HIV transmission during paediatric health care in sub-Saharan Africa: risks and evidence. *South African Medical Journal* 2004; 94: 109–116.

40. Reid S. Non-vertical HIV transmission in children in sub-Saharan Africa. *International Journal of STD & AIDS* 2009; 20: 820–827.

41. Okinyi M, Brewer DD, Potterat JJ. Horizontally acquired HIV infection in Kenyan and Swazi children. *International Journal of STD & AIDS* 2009; 20: 852–857.

42. Vaz P, Pedro A, Le Bozec S, Macassa E, Salvador S, Bibenfeld G, et al. Nonvertical, nonsexual transmission of human immunodeficiency virus in children. *Pediatric Infectious Diseases Journal* 2010; 29: 271–274.

43. Brewer DD. Scarification and male circumcision associated with HIV infection in Mozambican children and youth. *WebmedCentralEPIDEMIOLOGY* 2011, 2 (9); WMC002206. http://www.webmedcentral.com/article_view/2206

44. Brewer DD, Gisselquist D, Brody S, Potterat JJ. Investigating iatrogenic HIV transmission in Ugandan children. *Journal of Acquired Immune Deficiency Syndromes* 2007; 45: 253–254.

45. Gisselquist D, Upham G, Potterat JJ. Efficiency of human immunodeficiency virus transmission through medical procedures: evidence, estimates, and unfinished business. *Infection Control & Hospital Epidemiology* 2006; 27 (9): 944–952.

46. Walker PR, Worobey M, Rambaut A, Holmes EC, Pybus OG. Sexual transmission of HIV in Africa: other routes of infection are not the dominant contributor to the African epidemic. *Nature* 2003; 422: 679.

47. Potterat JJ, Brewer DD, Rothenberg RB, Muth SQ, Brody S. HIV and hepatitis C epidemics in Africa: continuing the debate. *AIDScience* 2003; 3: 19 (16 October).

48. Layden JE, Phillips RO, Owusu-Ofori, Sarfo FS, Kliethermes S, Mora N, et al. High frequency of active HCV infection among seropositive cases in West Africa and evidence for multiple transmission pathways. *Clinical Infectious Diseases* 2015; 60: 1033–1041.

49. Brody S, Potterat JJ. Assessing the role of anal intercourse in the epidemiology of AIDS in Africa. *International Journal of STD & AIDS* 2003; 14: 431–436.

50. Brody S, Potterat JJ. Establishing valid AIDS monitoring and research in countries with generalized epidemics. *International Journal of STD & AIDS* 2004; 15: 1–6.

51. Potterat JJ. Estimating female-to-male infectivity of HIV-1 in Kenya: potential threats to validity. *The Journal of Infectious Diseases* 2005; 191: 2154–2155.

52. Potterat JJ, Brody S, Brewer DD, Muth SQ. Assessing anal intercourse and blood exposures as routes of HIV transmission in Mombasa, Kenya. *Sexually Transmitted Infections* 2008; http://sti.bmj.com/cgi/eletters/sti.2007.028852v1

53. Brewer DD, Potterat JJ, Roberts JM Jr., Brody S. Male and female circumcision associated with prevalent HIV infection in virgins and adolescents in Kenya, Lesotho, and Tanzania. *Annals of Epidemiology* 2007; 17: 217–226.

54. Deuchert E, Brody S. The role of health care in the spread of HIV/AIDS in Africa: evidence from Kenya. *International Journal of STD & AIDS* 2006; 17: 749–752.

55. Deuchert E, Brody S. Lack of auto-disable syringe use and health care indicators are associated with high HIV prevalence: an international ecological analysis. *Annals of Epidemiology* 2007; 17: 199–207.

56. Deuchert E. Maternal health care and the spread of AIDS in Burkina Faso and Cameroon. *World Health Population* 2007; 9: 55–72.

57. Deuchert E, Brody S. Plausible and implausible parameters for mathematical modeling of nominal heterosexual transmission. *Annals of Epidemiology* 2007; 17: 237–244.

58. Gisselquist D, Friedman E, Potterat J, Minkin SF, Brody S. Four policies to reduce HIV transmission through health care. *International Journal of STD & AIDS* 2003; 14: 717–722.

59. Gisselquist D. Points to Consider: Responses to HIV/AIDS in Africa, Asia, and the Caribbean. London, Adonis & Abbey Publishers, 2007. (Updated version available free at http://davidgisselquist.googlepages.com/pointstoconsider)

60. Brewer DD. Knowledge of blood-borne transmission risk is inversely associated with HIV infection in sub-Saharan Africa. *The Journal of Infection in Developing Countries* 2011; 5: 182–198.

61. Gisselquist D, Potterat JJ, Salerno L. Injured and insulted: women in Africa suffer from incomplete messages about HIV risks. *Horn of Africa Journal of AIDS* 2007; 4 (1): 15–18. http://www.peoplepeople.org/index.php?P=47

62. Peters EJ, Immananagha KK, Essien OE, Ekott JU. Traditional healers' practices and the spread of HIV/AIDS in south eastern Nigeria. *Tropical Doctor* 2004; 34: 79–82.

63. Peters EJ, Brewer DD, Udonwa NE, Jombo GTA, Essien OE, Umoh VA, Otu AA, Eduwern DU, Potterat JJ. Diverse blood exposures associated with incident HIV infection in Calabar, Nigeria. *International Journal of STD & AIDS* 2009; 20: 846–851.

64. Brewer D, Okinyi M, Potterat J. The facts about HIV infected Swazi children. *Times of Swaziland* 2009 (16 December): http://www.times.co.sz/index.php?news=12942

65. St. Lawrence JS, Klaskala W, Kankasa C, West JT, Mitchell CD, Wood C. Factors associated with HIV prevalence in a post-partum cohort of Zambian women. *International Journal of STD & AIDS* 2006; 17: 607–613.

66. Reid S, Van Niekerk AA. Injection risks and HIV transmission in the Republic of South Africa. *International Journal of STD & AIDS* 2009; 20: 816–819.

67. Reid S, Dawad S, Van Niekerk AA. Iatrogenic HIV transmission in South Africa: evidence, estimates and moral perspectives. *South Africa Family Practice* 2010; 52: 476–477.

68. Reid S, Juma OA. Minimum infective dose of HIV for parenteral dosimetry. *International Journal of STD & AIDS* 2009; 20: 828–833.

69. Reid S. Increase in clinical prevalence of AIDS implies increase in unsafe medical injections. *International Journal of STD & AIDS* 2009; 20: 295–299.

70. Epstein H. The Invisible Cure: Africa, the West, and the Fight against AIDS. New York: Farrar, Strauss & Giroux, 2007.

71. Potterat JJ. Attractive theory is not enough. *International Journal of STD & AIDS* 2007; 18: 645–646.

72. Lurie MN, Rosenthal S. Concurrent partnerships as a driver of the HIV epidemic in sub-Saharan Africa? The evidence is limited. *AIDS Behavior* 2009; 14: 17–24.

73. Sawers L, Stillwaggon E. Concurrent sexual partnerships do not explain the HIV epidemics in Africa: a systematic review of the evidence. *Journal of the International AIDS Society* 2010; 13: 34.

74. Sawers L, Stillwaggon E, Hertz T. Cofactor infections and HIV epidemics in developing countries: implications for treatment. *AIDS Care* 2008; 20: 488–494.

75. Akeke VA, Mokgatle M, Oguntibeju OO. Tattooing and risk of transmitting HIV in Quthing prison, Lesotho. *International Journal of STD & AIDS* 2007; 18: 363–364.

76. Centers for Disease Control and Prevention. HIV among male inmates in a state prison system—Georgia, 1992–2005. *Morbidity and Mortality Weekly Report* 2006; 55: 421–426.

77. Apetrei C, Becker J, Metzger M, Gautam R, Engle J, Wales KA, et al. Potential for HIV transmission through unsafe injections. *AIDS* 2006; 20: 1074–1076.

78. Priddy F, Tesfaye F, Mengistu Y, Rothenberg R, Fitzmaurice D, Mariam DH, et al. Potential for medical transmission of HIV in Ethiopia. *AIDS* 2005; 19; 348–350.

79. Lopman BA, Garnett GP, Mason PR, Gregson S. Individual level injection history: a lack of association with HIV incidence in rural Zimbabwe. *Public Library of Science Medicine* 2005; 2: 37.

80. Buve A, Laga M. Epidemiological research in the HIV field: towards understanding what we do not know. *AIDS* 2012; 26: 1203–1204.

81. Hunsmann M. Political determinants of variable aetiologic resonance: explaining the African AIDS epidemics. *International Journal of STD & AIDS* 2009; 20: 834–838.

82. Gisselquist D. Double standards in research ethics, health-care safety, and scientific rigour allowed Africa's HIV/AIDS epidemic disasters. *International Journal of STD & AIDS* 2009; 20: 839–845.

83. Gisselquist D. Denialism undermines HIV prevention in sub-Saharan Africa. *International Journal of STD & AIDS* 2008; 19: 649–655.

84. Gisselquist D. HIV infections as unanticipated problems during medical research in Africa. *Accountability in Research* 2009; 16: 199–217.

85. Gisselquist D, Potterat JJ, St. Lawrence JS, Hogan M, Arora NK, Correa M, Dinsmore W, Mehta G, Millogo J, Muth SQ, Okinyi M, Ounga T. How to contain generalized HIV epidemics? A plea for better evidence to displace speculation. *International Journal of STD & AIDS 2009*; 20: 443–446.

86. Brewer DD, Potterat JJ, Muth SQ. Withholding access to research data. *The Lancet* 2010; 375: 1872.

87. Mapingure MP, Msuya S, Kurewa NE, Munjoma MW, Sam N, Chirenje MZ, et al. Sexual behavior does not reflect HIV-1 prevalence differences: a comparison study of Zimbabwe and Tanzania. *Journal of the International AIDS Society* 2010; 13: 45. doi: 10.1186/1758-2652-13-45.

88. Duri K, Stray-Pedersen B. HIV/AIDS in Africa: trends, missing links and the way forward. *Journal of Virology & Antiviral Research* 2013; 2: 1. doi.org/10.4172/2324-8955.1000107.

89. Kimani D, Kamau R, Ssempijja V, Robinson K, Oluoch T, Njeru M, et al. Medical injection use among adults and adolescents aged 15 to 64 years in Kenya: results from a national survey. *Journal of the Acquired Immune Deficiency Syndromes* 2014; 66 (Suppl. 1): S57–S65.

90. Gisselquist D, Potterat JJ. Review of evidence from risk factor analyses associating HIV infection in African adults with medical injections and multiple sexual partners. *International Journal of STD & AIDS* 2004; 15: 222–233.

91. Gisselquist D, Potterat JJ, Brody S, Minkin SF. Does selected ecologic evidence give a true picture of HIV transmission in Africa? *International Journal of STD & AIDS* 2004; 15: 434–439.

92. Gisselquist D, Potterat JJ, Brody S. Running on empty: sexual cofactors are insufficient to drive Africa's turbocharged HIV epidemic. *International Journal of STD & AIDS* 2004; 15: 442–452.

93. Rothenberg R, Gisselquist D, Potterat J. A simulation to assess the conditions required for high level heterosexual transmission in Africa. *International Journal of STD & AIDS* 2004; 15: 529–532.

94. Ndinya-Achola JO, Plummer FA, Ronald AR, Piot P. Acquired Immunodeficiency syndrome: epidemiology in Africa and its implications for health services. *African Journal of Sexually Transmitted Diseases* 1986; 2: 77–80.

95. Quinn TC, Mann JM, Curran JW, Piot P. AIDS in Africa: an epidemiologic paradigm. *Science* 1986; 234: 955–963.

96. Gisselquist D, Potterat JJ. Request for disclosure of available data associating HIV with medical injections. http://uqconnect.net/signfiles/Archives/SIGN-POST00269.txt (20 December 2004).

97. Sarewitz D. Beware the creeping cracks of bias. *Nature* 2012; 485: 149.

98. See: http://rationalwiki.org/wiki/Argument_from_adverse_consequences

99. Britton S. The HIV/AIDS pandemic: at last good news. *Scandinavian Journal of Public Health* 2004; 32: 3–5.

100. Mills EJ, Ford N. HIV status in serodiscordant couples (Authors' reply). *Lancet Infectious Diseases* 2011; 11: 658–659.

101. Fuller T. Shock and anger in Cambodian village struck with H.I.V. *The New York Times*, 20 January 2015, p. A4, A8.

EPILOGUE

1. Potterat JJ. Disease intervention specialists as a corps, not corpse. *Sexually Transmitted Diseases* 2008; 35: 703.

ACKNOWLEDGMENTS

Star players are part of a team. This certainly applies to each of the stars listed below. If they are highlighted it is because of their exceptional efforts and contributions to the Colorado Springs STD/HIV program over long periods. They are stars of very bright luminosity and no words suffice to express my deep and abiding appreciation for their sustained hard work and fierce loyalty.

Thank you…

…**Heavenly Boss:** John B. Muth MD MPH.

…**Contact Tracers Extraordinaire:** Dave Green, Lynanne Plummer Phillips RN, MPH, Christopher I. Pratts, Helen L. Zimmerman-Rogers, Jerry E. Taylor, and Donald E. Woodhouse MPA, JD.

…**STD Clinic Luminaries:** Jimmie Combs RN, James S. Fogle III MT, Esther M. Lackey MD, Gary S. Markewich MD, Judith U. Reynolds MD, Helen P. Zimmerman RN.

…**Data Systems Resident Savant and Able Assistant:** Stephen Q. Muth and Tammy S. Maldonado-Long.

…**Exceptional External Experts:** Devon D. Brewer, PhD, Stuart M. Brody PhD, William W. Darrow PhD, Alden S. Klovdahl PhD, Richard B. Rothenberg MD, MPH, Thomas M. Vernon MD, MPH.

Supporting Cast:

During the three decades (through year 2000) that I had the privilege of directing the STD/HIV control programs, many, many people provided short-term assistance and should be acknowledged and warmly thanked. I apologize to anyone whose name fails to appear or is misspelled—an artifact of both imperfect memory and lack of access to personnel records. Here is a reasonably complete list of part-timers and of support personnel kindly "loaned" from other health department sections, alphabetically:

Joanne Abair, Lauren Alt, Rajko Anic MD, Diane Ashton RN, Millie Baer RN, Gina Bamberger DO, Diane Bartok RN, Perry Bethea, Richard Blair, Mandy Bonney, Richard Borkow MD, Nancy Brace RN, Joe Brady, Corliss Brecht RN, Donald Bross JD, PhD, J. Richard Brusenhan MD, Patrick Carter DO, Opal Clark, Mike Cliett, Patricia Cox, W. B. Crouch MD, Beverley Dahan, Chris Dale, Rita Dawson, Daniel Depperman, Hal Dewlett MD, Joel Dickerman DO, Dayna Dorobiala, Charles Dowding Jr. MD, Andrea Dubose, Richard Dukes PhD, Harold Dyer MD, Evie Evans RN, Lani Fair, Carolyn Ferree RN, Sonya Garvin, Deanna Green MT, Jean Harris RN, Mary Haukom RN, Julie Higgins, Randy Hoffman DO, Beth Holtby RN, Shana Hurlbutt-Sanderson, Susan Janty RN, Jeanette Jaramillo, Franklyn Judson MD, Cheryl Justis, Michael King, Richard D. King MD, Tobias Kircher MD, Joyce Klinger MT, Helen Koons RN, Gloria Latimer, Frieda Laubach RN, Judy Leiseth, Mary Linthicum, Bill Lowe, Patsy McAteer RN,

Patricia Malone, Mary Martinez, Elizabeth Mattas, Joyce Michael DO, Pamela Montoya, Moonyin, Esther Morelli, Lee Norgaard, Robin Reed Nypaver RN, Lisa Otoupalik, Vicky Otoupalik-Huffor, Joy Peterson, Mike Plunkett, my daughter Anna Potterat, Pyper Prosen, Diane Richards, Edward Richards JD, Miche Rodolph, Mary Jo Rosazza RN, Sheryl Rose DO, Tauni Ryan NP, John Seay, R. Michael Sherwin MD, Charli Shumate, Linda Silveira DO, Nancy Spencer, Donald Spradlin DO, Sally Stark RN, Heather Stites, Janice Tolzman MLT, Trudy Tong, Barbara Trombley RN, Chris Urzinger, Ekaterina Walker MD, Maria Ward, George Ware, Helen White, Nancy Wilstead NP, Frederick Wolf, Jane Worrall MT, and Lynn Wright.

INDEX

ABOUT THE AUTHOR

John Potterat is one of the country's leading sexually transmissible diseases epidemiologists. He has devoted his professional life to STD/HIV control since 1968, first with the CDC's syphilis eradication program (1968–1972) and, subsequently (1972–2001), with the health department in Colorado Springs, where he focused on community STD/HIV transmission dynamics; on the configuration of sexual networks underlying gonorrhea, chlamydia, and HIV transmission; on contact tracing initiatives; and on the epidemiology of prostitution. He is currently an independent consultant specializing in the epidemiology of AIDS in Africa, with time to pursue his favorite hobbies: reading non-fiction, tennis, and collecting ancient coins. He is married—with grown, independent children—and lives with his wife Susan and Black Lab Emmy in Colorado Springs.

Website is: http://home.earthlink.net/~jjpotterat/

GOOGLE Scholar page: http://tinyurl.com/jwsre62

www.ingramcontent.com/pod-product-compliance
Lightning Source LLC
Chambersburg PA
CBHW051209170526
45166CB00005B/1819